Medicine and Religion

Medicine and Religion

A Historical Introduction

Gary B. Ferngren

Johns Hopkins University Press
Baltimore

© 2014 Johns Hopkins University Press
All rights reserved. Published 2014
Printed in the United States of America on acid-free paper

9 8 7 6 5 4 3 2 1

Johns Hopkins University Press
2715 North Charles Street
Baltimore, Maryland 21218-4363
www.press.jhu.edu

Library of Congress Cataloging-in-Publication Data

Ferngren, Gary B.
   Medicine and religion : a historical introduction / Gary B. Ferngren.
      pages cm
   Includes bibliographical references and index.
ISBN 978-1-4214-1215-3 (hardcover : alk. paper) — ISBN 978-1-4214-1216-0
(pbk. : alk. paper) — ISBN 978-1-4214-1217-7 (electronic) —
ISBN 1-4214-1215-2 (hardcover : alk. paper) — ISBN 1-4214-1216-0
(pbk. : alk. paper) — ISBN 1-4214-1217-9 (electronic)
   1. Medicine—Religious aspects.   I. Title.
BL65.M4F47 2014
201'.661—dc23   2013015237

A catalog record for this book is available from the British Library.

*Special discounts are available for bulk purchases of this book. For more informa-
tion, please contact Special Sales at 410-516-6936 or specialsales@press.jhu.edu.*

Johns Hopkins University Press uses environmentally friendly book materials,
including recycled text paper that is composed of at least 30 percent post-
consumer waste, whenever possible.

For my daughters
   Suzie Mancus
   Anne-Marie Nakhla
   Heather Morton
who so resemble their mother

Contents

Acknowledgments

Much of my research in the course of my academic career has been devoted to exploring the intersection of religion and medicine, for the most part but not exclusively in the ancient world. I received a traditional training in classics for the PhD, specializing in Greek and Roman history. While I did not study medical history in the course of my graduate training, I found it sufficiently interesting that early in my career I began to devote a good deal of time to the study of Greek medicine. My introduction to the subject came at an opportune time. The social history of medicine was attracting a good deal of attention from professional historians, and it rapidly became a growth industry. My research led to a series of studies on Greek and Greco-Roman medicine, many of them written in collaboration with my colleague Darrel Amundsen, of Western Washington University. My parallel interest in religion made it natural for me to focus my attention on the relationship of medicine to Greek religion before I broadened my research to include a study of early Christian approaches to medicine, healing, and philanthropic health care.

While there are many books that deal with medicine and religion and still more that explore or describe the broader subject of spirituality and healing, broad historical surveys of the subject are relatively uncommon. Some thirty years ago Darrel Amundsen and I collaborated on two chapters that traced the relationship between religion and medicine from the civilizations of the ancient Near East to the end of the Middle Ages. Since then much new scholarship, the result of the renaissance of interest in the history of medicine, has greatly extended our knowledge of what we described in those chapters. The present volume both incorporates that scholarship and carries forward the historical treatment to the modern age.

The reader should keep in mind that this book is neither a history of medicine nor a history of religion. The focus of the treatment and restrictions of space required that in both fields I omit much that would in another context be of interest, if not essential. I have not written a scholarly monograph but rather an introduction intended for nonspecialists who wish to gain an understanding of the place of religion in the Western medical and healing traditions. For that reason I have avoided arcane language and technical medical terms. I have kept annotation to a minimum and have confined the notes chiefly to citations rather than to extended discussions, a decision that I have revisited several times. Scholars will miss the linking of the narrative to primary and secondary texts. But providing the annotation to accomplish that desirable end would have increased the length of the volume to a point that would not have been economically viable. For each chapter an extensive bibliography of secondary literature on medicine and religion, with an emphasis on recent publications in English, is available at the publisher's website (www.press.jhu.edu); search for this book by title or by author for a link to the bibliography. These bibliographies will permit the reader to pursue subjects of special interest.

My purpose in this volume is to provide a concise but comprehensive survey that traces the history of the intersection of medicine and healing with religious traditions in the Western world from the earliest civilizations of Mesopotamia and Egypt to our own era. In chapters 1 to 8 I describe a range of healing and health-care issues within both the polytheistic belief systems of the ancient world and the monotheistic faiths of Judaism, Christianity, and Islam. Some readers will miss the inclusion of non-Western traditions, such as Shamanistic, Persian, Indian, African, and Chinese and other Asian medical traditions. Here the limits of my personal knowledge were paramount. I simply do not command the knowledge necessary to write on those traditions with confidence. The costs of publishing today, moreover, imposed constraints on the length of the book. For this reason I found it necessary to delete from my narrative an account of the development of psychology, psychiatry, and, to a lesser extent, medical ethics and their interaction with religion in the nineteenth and twentieth centuries. Because this volume is directed to a largely North American readership, my focus in chapter 8 is on American developments, movements, and personalities.

"Authors," write Peter and Linda Murray in their introduction to *The Oxford Companion to Christian Art and Architecture* (1996), "write with whatever abilities, knowledge, and perseverance they may possess, but it is upon the combined labours of a whole team that any successful outcome depends, and no author should ever forget it." I have not forgotten it. I am grateful for a residential fellowship that I held at the Oregon State University Center for the Humanities during the fall quarter of 2011. A grant from David Robinson, director of the center, permitted me to secure professional indexing for the volume. Chapter 6 was coauthored by Mahdieh Tavakol, whose expertise in an area with which I lack familiarity I am delighted to acknowledge. Earlier versions of portions of chapters 1, 2, and 5 were coauthored by Darrel Amundsen.

Because this volume covers a broad chronological sweep, I have largely depended on secondary rather than original sources for the periods in which I am not an expert. But I have invited experts in the field to read and critique each of the chapters to ensure their accuracy and balance. The following have given generously of their time in reading one or more of the chapters: Anne-Marie Nakhla (introduction); Daniel and Annette Youngberg (introduction and epilogue); Robert D. Biggs, the Reverend Martin Emmrich, Andrew Teeter, and Kent R. Weeks, each of whom read a portion of chapter 1; Ildikó Csepregi (chs. 2, 3, and 4); Charles Odahl (ch. 3); Luke Demaitre, Timothy Miller, John Riddle, Lisa Sarasohn, and Harry York (ch. 5); Jonathan Katz, Seyyed Hossein Nasr, and Ahmed Ragab (ch. 6); Anita Guerrini, Joel Klein, Ekaterina N. Lomperis, and Paul Kopperman (ch. 7); Darryl Hart, Aline Kalbian, Amy L. Koehlinger, and Ronald Numbers (ch. 8); and Darrel Amundsen (epilogue). Joy Abbott provided exceptionally efficient assistance in the preparation of the manuscript, as did Jane Yao in library research. Heather Morton improved the style and logic of several chapters. It is my pleasure once more to acknowledge the assistance of Jacqueline Wehmueller, Executive Editor of the Johns Hopkins University Press, who would be any author's idea of the perfect editor and who is certainly mine. I acknowledge as well the assistance of Linda Forlifer, Sarah J. Cleary, and Joanne Allen. I dedicate this volume to my daughters, Suzie Mancus, Anne-Marie Nakhla, and Heather Morton. Few fathers have had more loving and devoted daughters.

Portions of several chapters originally appeared elsewhere. I acknowledge permission to incorporate the following, in whole or in part, with many modifications and adaptations, into this volume:

"Medicine and Religion: Pre-Christian Antiquity" and "Medicine and Religion: Early Christianity through the Middle Ages" (both with Darrel W. Amundsen), in *Health/Medicine and the Faith Traditions: An Inquiry into Religion and Medicine*, edited by Martin E. Marty and Kenneth L. Vaux (Philadelphia: Fortress Press, 1982), 53–92 and 93–131. Reprinted in part with the permission of Advocate Lutheran General Hospital.

"The Evangelical-Fundamentalist Tradition," in *Caring and Curing: Health and Medicine in the Western Religious Traditions*, edited by Ronald L. Numbers and Darrel W. Amundsen (1986; reprint, Baltimore: Johns Hopkins University Press, 1997). Reprinted in part with the permission of Advocate Lutheran General Hospital.

"Galen" and "Hippocrates" (revised) in *Encyclopedia of Religion*, edited by Lindsay Jones, 2nd ed. (New York: Macmillan Reference, 2004), 5:3255–56 and 6:4021–22. Reprinted in part with the permission of Macmillan Reference.

"The Discourses of Protestant Medical Ethics," in *The Cambridge World History of Medical Ethics*, edited by Robert B. Baker and Laurence B. McCullough (New York: Cambridge University Press, 2009) 255–63. Portions reprinted with the permission of Cambridge University Press.

Medicine and Health Care in Early Christianity (Baltimore: Johns Hopkins University Press, 2009). Portions reprinted with the permission of Johns Hopkins University Press.

"History of Medicine (Western)," in *Encyclopedia of Sciences and Religions*, edited by Nina P. Azari (Dordrecht: Springer, 2013). Portions reprinted with the kind permission of Springer Science and Business Media.

"Medicine and Religion—A Historical Perspective," in *Oxford Textbook of Spirituality in Health Care*, edited by Mark Cobb, Christina Puchalski, and Bruce Rumfeld (Oxford: Oxford University Press, 2012). Portions reprinted with the permission of Oxford University Press.

Medicine and Religion

Introduction

When your mother is sick, or your child, do you pray or call the doctor? Is an infection attacking her body, or is there a spiritual issue to confront? For many who live in modern Western societies the very question is absurd. We are conditioned to see medicine as a purely biological or physical phenomenon. Those who pray instead of consulting their local physician we deem foolish and irresponsible. In some cases they are taken to court and sentenced to prison for their irresponsibility in not seeking medical care for their children. The more religiously minded among us might offer a prayer while driving to the hospital, asking the Divine Healer for help or wisdom. But it is the physician to whom we first bring our physical ailments and in whom we ultimately place our trust.

To the educated mind, the association of religion with healing seems an anachronism that is incompatible with scientific medicine. In fact, however, this attitude is a modern one that is informed by the naturalistic values that hold sway in intellectual and scientific circles today. Most societies throughout history have espoused a religious view of the world, and many today do as well. Religion for them encompasses the totality of life and is connected with every facet of existence, including healing. Medicine and religion have had a close association throughout history, one that can be traced back to the earliest human attempts to heal the human body and to understand the meaning of illness. In the ancient world, when little was known about theoretical medicine or the structure of the body, healers often treated the symptoms of common diseases, while the causes remained mysterious and were ascribed to vague or malignant spirits or to demons or divine beings, such as Apollo, who shot disease-bearing arrows at Greek armies, or the Roman spirit Febris (Fever). Experienced healers, moreover, knew their limitations. They treated many conditions for which there were no cures and turned more quickly than do moderns to supernatural forces for help. Those who practiced the healing arts understood that in cases where they could do little the best—and in some cases the only—hope of physical restoration came from the gods.

Even today the religious beliefs of many Westerners intersect with the culture of healing and health care in surprisingly traditional ways. These beliefs often lie under the radar of public or media perception and, when made public, may be ridiculed as hopelessly anachronistic. Yet a belief in God often quietly motivates a physician or health-care worker to provide compassionate care for those who are ill, or to help the sick endure pain and suffering, or to give spiritual consolation to the dying. Physicians and patients alike pray for divine help and healing, especially when they have exhausted all the avenues of modern science and medical knowledge. Faith today still offers the hope of some relief to many who experience chronic or untreatable diseases. And it provides a comfort that modern medicine and science do not: the belief that there is divine purpose in suffering, some meaning in all the pain one bears. Perhaps faith even holds a role in healing not altogether foreign to that of the ancient world, although modern men and women might take quite a few steps along their medical journey before realizing that they may have need of their faith before that journey is over.

The Historiography of Religion and Medicine

It is difficult for us, living in an age in which medicine is driven by intensive research and technological innovation, to appreciate or even understand premodern medicine. Take, for example, phlebotomy, or bloodletting, which was commonly used by physicians as late as the early nineteenth century. George Washington's death was hastened by physicians who relieved his weak body of too much blood.[1] The practice sounds primitive to modern ears, yet it was a rational procedure based on the acceptance of humoral pathology, according to which health was the result of the balance of the body's humors (fluids). The blood was believed to contain all four humors, any one of which could become a harmful matter that needed to be drawn off to restore health. Reducing the corrupt humor was thought to bring about recovery. A procedure that may strike us as repugnant becomes slightly less so once we understand the historical context in which it was practiced.

In the past generation, historical scholarship has devoted a good deal of attention to the relationship between science and religion. Two recent influential historiographic perspectives provide the orientation of this book. The first is the reaction against what is commonly called *Whiggism*. The term denotes a perspective that views the past through the lens of the present and sees history as moving progressively toward the ideas and institutions of a later age, particularly our own. It valorizes modern assumptions and can at times appear smug or triumphalist. Many historians of medicine writing today attempt to avoid the correlatives of Whiggism, namely, presentism and essentialism, which have often influenced the historical understanding of both religion and medicine. *Presentism* is the tendency to shape the past by employing modern definitions and understandings. It sometimes leads to the common practice of reading modern theories or discoveries back into the medical cultures of the past to demonstrate how far ahead they were of their own time and how close they were to modern ideas. *Essentialism* is the view that an idea or a discipline is basically the same in all ages. It is not uncommon for modern students of history to take medical concepts discussed in ancient texts to mean the same things we mean by them today; hence they use modern scientific terminology to translate ancient ideas that are grounded in—and limited by—their own cultural understanding.[2] By contrast, most contemporary historians believe that we distort the history of medicine by imposing modern definitions on the study of the past or by admitting as scientific only what a modern medical scientist would regard as such. Most medical practitioners throughout history have embraced one or more approaches to healing, whether theoretical or clinical, that would be regarded as unscientific by medical practitioners of today but were not regarded as such by the medical standards of their own time. I shall attempt to avoid the presentist and essentialist fallacies in favor of *contextualism*, an approach that recognizes that all medical ideas and practices, including our own, are shaped by their cultural context.

The second historiographic perspective that underlies this book is the rejection of the notion that there has existed throughout history an essential conflict between religion and science. The Draper-White, or "conflict," thesis was enormously influential in America at both popular and academic levels during much of the twentieth century. It has dominated historical interpretations of the relation between religion and science. John William Draper and Andrew Dickson White believed that Christianity had had a long history of opposing scientific progress. White, the first president of Cornell University, argued that the early church had hindered the progress of science and medicine both by denigrating the investigation of nature and by subordinating observation and reasoning to the authority of scripture and theology. As a result of this view, myths about the alleged hostility of Christianity to medicine have enjoyed wide currency. One such myth is that Christianity was responsible for the decline of ancient science. Another is that Christians opposed the use of anesthetics because they believed that it was wrong to relieve pain, which was the result of God's curse after the Fall. Yet another is that Christians were opposed to vaccination because they believed that it interfered with God's providential order. All have been disproved.[3]

In the late twentieth century the Draper-White thesis underwent a systematic reevaluation. Several contemporary historians of science and medicine (e.g., John Brooke, Ronald Numbers, and David Lindberg) have argued that relations between religion and science have been much more positive than is usually thought and often presented. John Brooke, in *Science and Religion: Some Historical Perspectives* (1991), suggests that a "complexity thesis," which views science and religion in a variety of relationships, some harmonious and some conflictive, is a more accurate model than the familiar conflict thesis. Recent studies have shown that Christianity has often nurtured and encouraged scientific and medical endeavors, while at other times the two have coexisted without either tension or attempts at harmonization. Christian clergymen, for example, actively supported the introduction of inoculation and anesthesia against the advice of many in the medical profession. Such a clergyman was the eighteenth-century Protestant minister Cotton Mather. Living in Boston during a smallpox epidemic, Mather actively supported vaccination in opposition to many of the town's doctors.

Tensions in Medicine and Religion

If one rejects the conflict model as simplistic in describing the relationship between medicine and religion, one can nevertheless observe tensions that historically have existed between the two. These are best seen by examining the various ways in which they have interacted. Darrel Amundsen has suggested that religion and medicine have been related in four different configurations throughout history.[4]

In the first, medicine has been subsumed under religion. In this model society is monolithic and there exists a single religious culture that is most often animistic or monistic, as in prehistoric or tribal cultures. Disease is viewed through a magico-religious lens, and therapy is administered by a shaman or religious person. A variant of this model occurs when a religiously homogeneous society attempts to fit medicine, even naturalistic medicine, into the prevailing religious framework. This was characteristic, for example, of the European Middle Ages, whose culture was very different from that of a tribal society but one that sought to understand medicine through a consistent religious world-view. A second variant may be found in those cases in which a religious minority in a pluralistic culture limits its community to a particular kind of healing that is at odds with the model of healing adopted by the larger culture. Healing sects throughout Western history have often fit this model, going against the grain by practicing religious or supernatural healing, while the larger culture sought healing by medicine.

A second model, according to Amundsen's typology, is one in which medicine and religion are partially separated. Societies of this kind understand disease naturalistically and employ rational or empirical medicine for healing. At the same time there exists some overlap between religion and medicine, particularly in societal values. This model was operative in classical Greece as well as in much of European history. In the latter, Judeo-Christian values, though challenged by the eighteenth-century Enlightenment, dominated Western societal values until the latter half of the twentieth century, particularly (as it related to medicine) in medical ethics.

A third model is one in which religion and medicine have become completely separated and compartmentalized. This is the situation in which we find ourselves today, one in which Western societies are both pluralistic and lacking a moral or religious consensus. This model is prone to tension because many religious adherents believe that a specific set of moral values ought to inform medicine, especially in the area of medical ethics, while those who wish to maintain religious neutrality are equally adamant that they should not. Many of the most polarizing issues of the early twenty-first century, such as abortion, euthanasia, and assisted suicide, have become battlegrounds for the adherents of these two points of view.

The fourth model is one in which religion is subsumed under medicine. Society develops a therapeutic approach to many health-related issues that previously would have been considered to fall at least partially within the domain of religion, such as aspects of mental health, social well-being, sex, and marriage and family relationships. In our own day even spirituality has come to be viewed within a therapeutic framework, one in which counselors replace pastors, while the language becomes one of developing a healthy physical and spiritual lifestyle and restoring one's harmony with nature. While the model is attractive in its appeal to nonsectarian categories, it too creates tensions, as traditional religious adherents view it as one in which faith is swallowed up by medicine cloaked in pseudo-religious dress.

In these four configurations the potential exists for inevitable tension, not because religion seeks to go beyond its boundaries in encroaching upon medicine (although in the first model the two are intertwined) but because the issue is one of defining the boundaries between medicine and religion. To medical practitioners in our own age, anxious to protect the gains of scientific medicine, any religious scruples regarding medical procedures is sometimes viewed as the resurgence of an antiquated world-view that challenges the claims of science. To the adherents of a religious point of view, medicine, like all human activities, should be informed by a moral framework and not merely by technological or material factors. The issues are perennial, but they do not represent simply another version of the alleged conflict between science and religion. Rather, they are two domains, each with its legitimate perspective, which have overlapping concerns.

Concepts of Health and Disease

Let us define *medicine* more specifically, since we will be contrasting it with religion consistently throughout this book. Medicine, as we will use the term, is the art of preserving or restoring health and treating disease, illness, or physical disability by means of drugs, surgical procedures, or physical manipulations. What of *religion*? Perhaps the *Oxford English Dictionary*'s is as close as one can find to a general definition that includes both theistic and less defined forms, such as Buddhism and Hinduism. According to the *OED*, religion is the "recognition on the part of man of some higher unseen power as having control of his destiny, and as being entitled to obedience, reverence, and worship."[5] The history of medicine is the history of both changing concepts of health and disease and the greatly varied social roles and ethical responsibilities of those who seek to preserve or restore health. The impact of religion on the history of medicine in its broadest sense as well as in some of its specific disciplines is reflected in the history of those changing concepts. The roles and responsibilities of medical practitioners, while affected by changing scientific ideas, are less features of the history of science than of social and cultural history.

The current study of the history of medicine has tended to emphasize contextualism over the earlier dominance of Whiggism. A contextual approach examines history in terms of its cultural context, without attention to where its ideas have led and therefore whether they accord with modern views. While grounding medical practice and ideas in their own culture, this approach makes it more difficult to provide precise definitions of key terms in the history of medicine.

Indeed, contemporary writing in the field tends to avoid general definitions in favor of carefully nuanced and temporally conditioned conceptualizations. An example is found in the variety of definitions of health that have been given at different times and in different cultures. *Health* is an imprecise term. While its basic definition is the absence of disease, words for *health* in many languages are semantically related to ideas of physical wholeness and are virtually synonymous with *wellness* and even *well-being*. They seek to describe a balanced personality in which mind, body, and spirit are in harmony. The best-known modern definition is that of the World Health Organization, which defines health as a "state of complete physical, mental, and social well-being, and not merely the absence of disease or infirmity." This broad concept, which is grounded in Enlightenment assumptions, appears to make health nearly indistinguishable from human happiness.

Every language employs a variety of words, some precise and some imprecise, to express physical disability and dysfunction. The spectrum of disease includes sickness, infirmity, illness, mild physical discomfort, and deformity. *Disease*, like *health*, can be used metaphorically and applied to body, mind, and soul. The term *disease* is as malleable as *health,* as can be seen in its application to such cultural "diseases" as alcoholism. When imprecise terms are used to indicate that someone is ill, the language is usually not scientific and does not denote a particular medical condition. One often employs general terms to express merely the perception that one is not, in the commonly accepted understanding of the term, in good health. Hence words like *illness* and *sickness* carry with them a social or cultural rather than a scientific medical connotation, as in "I feel ill." Among medical anthropologists *disease* is usually taken to describe a biological entity, while *illness* denotes a subjective feeling of physical discomfort. One might say that disease is the objective, illness the subjective, component. But even when one employs a specific or medical vocabulary, if it is symptomatic rather than pathological it normally reflects the particular culture that created it rather than a scientific description. And when the vocabulary of disease becomes pathologically precise, it reflects a particular medical model that is culture-specific and cannot be taken as necessarily consistent with modern medical constructs.

This point can be illustrated by medical terms taken from almost any nonmedical text written by laypersons in the classical world of Greece and Rome. The New Testament Gospels provide us with a familiar example. They sometimes describe a person as having a pathological condition, such as fever or dysentery, or as suffering from a congenital condition, such as being crippled or having a

flow of blood, or as having leprosy or being moonstruck (i.e., struck with lu-
nacy). In these instances there is no certain method for determining precisely
which condition is being related, and so it is difficult to convert them into contemporary medical models or pathologies. When the terminology is imprecise
or generic—that is, when a person is described as sick, or faint, or possessed
of a fever—the problem is even more difficult. Such vocabulary almost always
denotes a lay description that is so medically imprecise as to be almost useless as
evidence for any specific medical condition. But even when disease is described
using the vocabulary of the humoral pathology of the classical world, the modern
reader faces the problem of translating the concept of one medical model into
another. The description might be a medical or scientific one, but it is likely to be
incompatible with a modern biomedical understanding of disease.

In general most nonmedical writers describe sickness and disease from the
point of view of external symptoms rather than in medical terms. Their non-
specialized vocabulary reflects an unscientific understanding of the physical
symptoms. Hence we will probably never know the precise pathological nature of
many of the diseases they describe. In the classical world *fever* was a generic term
that denoted a variety of infectious diseases that produced a high temperature,
while today it denotes only a symptom. This was true as well of jaundice, dropsy,
and asthma. The relation of a group of symptoms to a specific disease or disease
agent is a recent medical concept. Greek medical authors regarded diseases not
as separate entities but as groupings of symptoms that affected individuals and
could be described and classified. Many diseases that today are known to have a
specific cause were viewed differently in past societies. Today's syphilis first appeared in Europe in the late fifteenth century as the "Great Pox" or "the French
Disease" (*Morbus Gallicus*).[6] Hence modern medicine is not always very helpful
in providing either the physiological context or the tools for understanding the
nature of much of the disease described in premodern texts.

Modern studies of diseases found in earlier texts sometimes apply retrospective diagnosis, making identifications that impose a contemporary understanding of disease on the ancient writers. In fact, the modern interpreter who wishes
to determine the exact nature of ancient diseases faces intractable problems, beginning with the absence of semantic precision in the medical vocabulary and
the lack of medical clarity in describing symptoms, since many accounts, even
some medical texts, are lay narratives. Moreover, many descriptions of disease
are culture-specific. These problems are compounded by the chasm that separates historical and modern understandings of disease.

Many common diseases share so many similar features that we cannot identify them simply by their symptoms. It was only in the late nineteenth century that typhoid fever was recognized as a separate disease from typhus. Moreover, the symptoms and impact of a disease can vary with nutritional conditions and diet. Epidemics are rarely limited to a single disease. The Plague of Athens (430–429 BC) consisted of two distinct diseases, and the Black Death (1349–51), three. Finally, and perhaps most importantly, disease entities can and often do change altogether as they adapt by mutation over time to new hosts in altering environments. It is likely that many diseases have been transformed over the centuries and that the diseases that constituted the Plague of Athens cannot be precisely identified with any disease that exists today.

Healing

In antiquity and indeed up to the present, people have sought healing in different ways, most commonly by natural, religious, or magical means. Natural healing has ranged from the medicine of a physician to folk remedies, home cures, traditional treatments, and herbal recipes. Such folk or popular medicine has been found in every culture, ancient and modern, and has likely been the most usual means of treating illness in every age and society. It is based on traditional remedies that are transmitted by ordinary people from generation to generation and often relies on empirical treatments, including common-sense remedies with which most people were raised. Many of us know of medically untrained laypeople who seem to have an uncanny ability to diagnose their family's or friends' medical problems, perhaps intuitively, and to recommend a remedy. Some folk remedies are efficacious, while many are not. Their ability to heal depends on experience that is transmitted sometimes over centuries, with the remedies finding their way into both popular medical culture and handbooks of medical lore. There is nothing out of date about these remedies, since they are seldom influenced by advances in medicine or even by revolutions in medical theory.

Religious or divine healing, which is broader than what we often call "miraculous healing," seeks the assistance or the intervention of a divine power that transcends the normal course of nature. In the classical world of Greece and Rome *nature* (Gk., *phusis*; L., *natura*) referred to what could be known from ordinary human experience. Hence the Greeks understood human nature based on long-recognized and frequently observed behavior. Extraordinary behavior was behavior that was contrary to nature. In Greek medicine *hygieia* (health) was the term used to describe the normal condition of the body, while *nosos* (illness) denoted a departure from nature. Physicians attempted through treatment to restore the body to its natural state by an art that took its model from nature. When treatment failed, the patient might seek divine healing, which went beyond ordinary means, that is, beyond the medical art. The classical world understood patterns of frequency and regularity in nature and used them as a basis for recognizing exceptional phenomena. These categories were not limited to the learned, since ordinary people understood how nature worked, not in a theoretical sense but from personal observation. Some phenomena transcended their everyday experience: they were either extraordinary or inexplicable. Such phenomena did not necessarily involve supernatural intervention and were not always given explanation, but they did provoke awe and wonder and were regarded as marvelous. The understanding of how nature works varied from place to place and age to age, differing according to people's status and education. Yet it often transcended cultural, national, and religious differences. Belief in the possibility of divine intervention in nature was nearly universal in antiquity and has remained so, with some exceptions, throughout most periods of history, even in modern societies that have been influenced by naturalistic thinking. While the form and manner of miraculous healing have varied considerably, in the twenty-first century traditional healing sites such as Lourdes, Fatima, and Guadalupe continue to draw millions of pilgrims each year, and many Christians believe that they have experienced it.

A third means of healing is through magic, which involves the employment of amulets, incantations, and occult objects, such as herbs and gems that manipulate hidden preternatural forces within nature but outside its normal course. Many people have used a variety of magical or nonrational methods to complement medical treatment, regarding them all as legitimate and none as disreputable. While it is easy for the modern mind to regard the widespread use of magic for healing in earlier cultures with skepticism or amusement, every age, including our own, has employed it. The use of amulets or charms remains common today, from Saint Christopher medals to copper bracelets that are worn even by people of determined secular convictions. Amulets were—and are—believed to have special powers that either were apotropaic (preventive) or possessed the ability to heal. They were usually hung around the neck or attached to limbs. They often consisted of precious stones or herbs, sometimes even of animal parts. Closely related were incantations, which were magical texts that could be recited for healing purposes or to prevent demonic forces from entering the body. Sometimes they were inscribed in texts on precious stones or papyrus and worn as amulets. One finds them as early as Mesopotamian times.

It is nearly impossible to separate fully the three categories. They have repeatedly overlapped, and none has necessarily been thought incompatible with the others. All have been used for healing in the ancient and modern worlds, and the lines between them were sometimes as blurred in the ancient sources as they are in the minds of modern scholars. Hence the necessity to avoid rigidly imposing modern categories on the data that one finds in the primary texts or drawing neat but unhistorical distinctions between the three categories.

Therapeutic Efficacy and Patterns of Resort

Given the variety of definitions of health and disease in different cultures over several millennia, it is natural to wonder to what extent the widely different forms of therapy have achieved their purpose. It is doubtful whether a sick person gained much biomedical advantage from seeing a physician until less than two centuries ago. And much of the religious and magical therapy of traditional societies would be regarded today as superstition. The issue, however, is not whether premodern therapies were efficacious, that is, whether they genuinely healed disease; it is whether their recipients believed they did. In every society those suffering illness have sought medical care from practitioners who they believed could heal them, whether they offered natural, religious, or magical therapy. In fact, therapy of any age is self-authenticating if sufferers correlate it with the remission of their symptoms. Most diseases are self-limiting and end either in spontaneous remission or in death. Many symptoms of disease, even recurrent ones, are transient and respond to treatment. Two exceptions are chronic conditions, which are difficult to treat successfully, and epidemic diseases. No matter how limited or misguided a treatment may have been from a modern biomedical perspective, those who sought it expected to benefit from it and often did so. We call this benefit of anyone who seeks treatment for a medical condition *hoped-for results*. But healing also produces *expected results*. The healer or the therapy employed persuades the sufferer that it is a reasonable and valid approach to healing. Even if it does not produce hoped-for results, that is, even if the patient does not improve or live, the personal and professional authority of the healer and the treatment offered persuade the patient that it is an appropriate procedure even when it is overwhelmed by circumstances beyond the control of the healer. Moreover, because the therapy offered reflects the level of the culture and the moral and cosmological assumptions of the society that produced it, it provides an assurance that the attempt to restore health or reduce pain is in harmony with the world-view of the sufferer.[7]

But, one might ask, can primitive or premodern traditions of healing have been successful in healing disease? Can a procedure (e.g., phlebotomy) that is based on a mistaken understanding of the body (e.g., the humoral theory of disease) have commended itself to those suffering from illness? In answering the question, we must rid ourselves of the natural tendency to judge the past by present standards. Just as most people in a Western society like our own seek treatment from a medically trained physician, so most sufferers throughout history have sought treatment from the authoritative healers of their day. Since the time of Hippocrates, in fifth-century Greece, those who could afford treatment from a physician who accepted a natural understanding of disease sought medical aid that relied on natural treatment. But their ability to gain access to a physician depended on several contingencies, such as, for example, whether they lived in a city, where doctors might be easily found, or in a village or rural area, where they might not. Those who could not afford a physician's treatment sought aid from a variety of alternative healers, from folk practitioners to wise women, from root cutters to magicians. If they could not gain help from one group of healers, they sought help from another. One such possibility was the supernatural healing offered in temples of the healing god Asclepius, which by the second century AD could be found in hundreds of cities throughout the Roman Empire. We call this tendency of sufferers to seek healing from a variety of healers *patterns of resort*. In every generation the sick seek help wherever they can find it. This has been true especially of those experiencing chronic (long-term) pain. Sufferers from rheumatoid arthritis might seek help first from physicians, then from a variety of forms of alternative medicine, such as copper bracelets, uranium mines, and dietary remedies. Failing to find relief from one after another healer, they seek help from whatever sources offer some relief, no matter how problematic they are. Today the individual often exhausts the resources of the medical profession before going to alternative healers. Some travel to a religious healing site where sufferers have reported being healed by a saint or by the Virgin Mary. Some travel long distances to find healing by exotic means, either natural or preternatural, including shamanistic healers. This pattern has persisted over many centuries, and although the means of healing differ from age to age, a number of them are surprisingly similar. There is a correlation, moreover, between the expectation of an individual that he or she will be healed and the experience of being healed.

Conclusion

An imaginative gulf separates the medical world of previous historical ages from the modern world of advanced technology and sophisticated biomedicine. This gulf has a tendency to render us unconsciously patronizing toward earlier cultures that struggled with the same problems that confront us in a medical crisis: how to alleviate or learn to live with our own pain and suffering; how to account for our illnesses by placing them in a meaningful context or a broader framework that depends on nonmedical categories for understanding; and how to respond to the suffering of those around us. Earlier societies than ours faced similar issues and responded in similar ways. Their response more often than not involved religious answers to many of the questions they asked. To consider religious ritual, prayer, and vows a primitive approach to health and medicine is to be both presentist and unhistorical. Religion often gives answers that go beyond the realm of reason and logic, which are necessary but insufficient components of our self-awareness. "The heart has its reasons," wrote Pascal, "which reason does not know."[8] The history of the intersection of religion and medicine does not provide us with ready-made solutions to contemporary problems, but it does provide a broader context than do our more exclusively scientific categories for understanding the complexity of illness and suffering. And with that context comes a perspective that is often helpful as we struggle in confronting illness to make sense of some of life's most challenging issues.

Chapter One

The Ancient Near East

M esopotamia is a Greek word that means "the land between the rivers." It is the modern country of Iraq, which is bounded on the east by the Tigris River and on the west by the Euphrates. In ancient times it was divided into two parts. The northern half was called Assyria, the southern half Babylonia. Babylonia was in turn divided into Akkad in the north and Sumer in the south. At various times in history each of these regions dominated Mesopotamia. Hence the terms *Babylonia* and *Mesopotamia* are often used interchangeably.

Mesopotamia has sometimes been called the "cradle of civilization" because it was there that the components that make up civilization came together for the first time. A civilization may be defined as an advanced culture that is based on city life. Without the existence of cities, civilized life is impossible. During the Neolithic Revolution, which occurred in the Middle East as a gradual process between c. 9000 and c. 5000 BC, humans abandoned a nomadic life of hunting and gathering to live in villages, raise crops, and keep herds. As a result of this agricultural revolution, villages sprang up in many places throughout the Levant, Anatolia, and Mesopotamia. In the fourth millennium walled cities began to appear in Mesopotamia. About 3500 BC the Sumerians settled in the southern region (Sumer), and by c. 3200 BC they had invented the world's first writing system.

It is the invention of writing that separates prehistory (or preliterate history) from history, for writing permits the recording of historical events. The Sumerians wrote in *cuneiform*, a wedge-shaped script that was inscribed using a stylus on damp clay tablets, which were baked in the fierce heat of the Iraqi sun.[1] Cuneiform writing was used in Mesopotamia by the successive peoples (Akkadians, Amorites, Kassites, Assyrians) who established their dominance in the area and assimilated Sumerian civilization, which they transmitted until the conquest of Babylon in 539 BC ended forever the political supremacy of Babylonia and Assyria. It is in the cuneiform writings of the Mesopotamians, discovered by archaeologists in the palace archives of Mesopotamian kings, that we find our first recorded references to medicine and the medical art.

Both Egyptians and Mesopotamians lived under an absolute and despotic but sometimes benevolent monarchy. The king was the source of political authority and tied together all facets of life. Kingship was founded on and justified by a religious system that permeated society. In Egypt and Mesopotamia every aspect of life was molded by religion. All activities, including commercial and economic ones, depended upon the gods. The two spheres, human and divine, were brought together by the king, who in Egypt was a god descended among humans but in Mesopotamia was a human being who mediated between the two spheres. Herein lies a major difference between the Egyptian and Mesopotamian attitudes toward life. Mesopotamian culture was characterized by anxiety, uncertainty, and fear that the divine will might not be comprehended, to the harm or destruction of those seeking it. Thus the harmony of the two spheres was marred by a fear that the cosmic order, and hence the social order that depended on it, might at any time fall prey to chaos. Egypt, by contrast, was marked by constant serenity and happy resignation to the predestined order, because, with the pharaoh a god, the divine order (*ma'at*) was always knowable.

Both Egyptian and Mesopotamian religions were naturalistic and polytheistic, based on the worship of personified cosmic forces. The supreme good in life was harmony with the divine order in an unbroken relationship between humans and an animated nature. The inhabitants of the land felt secure only when they saw themselves at peace with the transcendent world. As the maintenance of this relationship was their responsibility, they expended much energy in attempting to preserve and, when necessary, restore that harmony between themselves and the gods. The religious world-view of these societies was steeped in magic. Injury and especially illness created disharmony, a dissonance between humans and their total environment. Although in the case of injury one might turn to the supernatural in seeking to understand why an accident or assault occurred, the immediate cause would be readily evident. What was not certain was the divine cause of sickness. As with the earliest human societies generally, so also with Egyptians and Mesopotamians, disease was usually viewed etiologically rather than symptomatically, that is, in a search for the beings who had brought about an illness.

In both Mesopotamia and Egypt the supernatural authors of disease were the gods, the dead, or demons. In Sumer, before the Akkadian conquest (c. 2350 BC) it was held that demons might attack through sorcery or as agents to bring about the fate of the afflicted or acted simply at random. Spirit intrusion was both the cause and the disease itself, and the intruding spirit was the morbid (diseased) element residing in the patient. The intruding spirit must be removed, but first it must be identified and the reason for its intrusion discerned by diagnosis. Mesopotamians believed that demons were ever present, and they lived in constant fear of being entered by a demon, which might bring death or disease. Amulets with a demon depicted on one side and an incantation on the other constituted a common prophylactic (disease-preventing) device against demonic intrusion.[2]

Purgatives (cathartics), which were frequently used in prescriptions, may have been intended to expel demons. Other causes of illness were the gods or ghosts of persons who had not been buried properly or who had died an unnatural death. When a god was diagnosed as being responsible for a disease, the sufferer would seek the assistance of the great gods indirectly. He would petition his own personal god, a minor deity who was seen as particularly interested in the man or his family. The personal gods, of whom there were many, could intercede with the great gods on behalf of their special devotees.

Some centuries after the Akkadian conquest two significant changes began to take place in Mesopotamian religion. First, the personal gods were viewed as more powerful than the demons and hence able to thwart their designs. Second, a conviction grew that illness was divine retribution for mistakes, failings, and ultimately sins in a sense not seen distinctly in Egyptian sources. If a demon succeeded in entering a man, it was because his personal god had turned away and permitted it to happen. Punitive illnesses sent by the gods could usually be removed only by the gods who had inflicted them. A god might punish a person for a variety of offenses, many of which were simply cultic or ritual violations that had no discernible moral overtones. The link between moral failing and retributive disease appears not to have been present in Egypt to the same degree that it was in Mesopotamia, where there was a much stronger sense of sin as a moral failing that precipitated divine retribution. Hence confessions constituted an important feature of therapy, often containing a formulaic statement such as, "My misdeeds are numerous; I have transgressed in every way." There existed in Mesopotamia over the centuries an increasing sensitivity to moral probity, as evidenced, for example, in the "mirror of confession," which listed a wide variety of sins ranging from disrespect of parents to abuse of the weak. The linking of sickness and sins was exploited in the Code of Hammurabi, in which Ninkarrak, a goddess of healing, is mentioned as inflicting sickness on those who do not obey the law.

Mesopotamia and Babylonia

In ancient Mesopotamia medicine and magic were equally legitimate in therapy, and the two were used in tandem. Medicine initially grew out of herbal remedies for sickness: plants, minerals, and animals or their products that could be ingested or inserted into the body or applied to its surface. Herbal remedies were commonly used to treat diseases of the skin, gastrointestinal problems, or respiratory problems, which were the most common complaints of those who sought medical help. Some herbal remedies were considered efficacious because healers had concluded from their own experience or from a long tradition of empirical observation that they accomplished the healing of certain illnesses. We have letters written by both physicians and their patients testifying to the apparent healing properties of certain herbals. We can never know, of course, whether the patient would have recovered without the prescription. Although many remedies were not efficacious, the patient may have considered them so. Of equal importance with medicine in Mesopotamia was the use of magic. While most modern readers consider magic either ineffectual or malign, in many instances it may have had a placebo effect that aided in healing.[3]

There were two distinct but complementary kinds of healers in Mesopotamia, the *āšipu* and the *asû*. The *āšipu*, who was always a man, was a magician and exorcist as well as a priest, while the *asû* was closer to what we would call a physician. The two did not stand in opposition to each other, nor do they appear to have been competitive rivals. The *āšipu* was concerned with diagnosis (the process of identifying a disease) and prognosis (forecasting its course). The *āšipu* attempted to identify the demon or determine the intentions of the god who had caused the illness and to indicate whether the illness was fatal or, if not, how long it would last. This was not always an easy task, since the Mesopotamian catalog of diseases listed some six thousand evil spirits who could cause disease. In complicated cases the *āšipu* recited a long list of possible sins to the patient in the hope that he or she might be able to choose from this list the offense that had produced his disease. If both methods failed, the *āšipu* had to resort to divination, for which he sometimes sought the aid of a *bārû* (diviner). He might practice many differ-ent kinds of divination, which was the art of discovering the future or discerning hidden knowledge. Astrology was the most important, but *hepatoscopy* (divining the disease from the shape and consistency of the liver of a sacrificial animal) was common as well. The liver was regarded as the body's main organ, produc-ing the blood that made life possible. Clay models of a sheep's liver were used to teach novices how to interpret them. Dreams were also used for divination, as were prodigies (abnormal births of humans and animals, whose interpretation is termed *teratology*) and the flight of birds.

In making his diagnosis the *āšipu* frequently consulted texts that contained sections on symptoms, etiology (the cause of a disease), diagnosis, and prognosis. If the prognosis was unfavorable, he would withdraw from the case. He used few if any drugs but quite reasonably attempted to cure through prayers and liba-tions. Treatment was strongly influenced by religious concepts. Confession, sac-rifice, and prayers were necessary to appease those gods who the Mesopotamians thought were angry at the patient. The incantations usually involved Gula, the Babylonian goddess of healing (one of her epithets was "Great Physician"), or Damu, a god of healing. Hundreds of texts of incantations survive from as early as the middle of the third millennium BC. The *āšipu* often recited them several times, although the patient was sometimes told to recite them instead.

Distinct from the *āšipu* was the *asû*, who was not a priest. He or she (there were some female physicians in Mesopotamia) was basically a craftsperson, al-though the treatment administered was not entirely devoid of magic in that the *asû* sometimes used incantations as an aid to treatment. In this there seems to have been a borrowing from the *āšipu*, although the inverse appears not to have been true. The therapeutic (healing) technique of the *asû* was an independent tradition that may have had its roots in an earlier, more primitive stage of sha-manism. But in Mesopotamia the procedures of the *asû* were functionally—if not always ideologically—separate from magico-religious procedures. Whereas the *āšipu* was concerned with etiology, the *asû* focused on therapy directed toward the relief of acute and pressing symptoms. Several lines from a hymn in which the goddess Gula, the Great Physician, praises herself provide a fine description of the profession of the *asû*:

> I am a physician, I can heal,
> I carry around all (healing) herbs, I drive away disease
> I gird myself with the leather bag containing health-giving incantations.

I carry around texts which bring recovery,
I give cures to mankind.
My pure dressing alleviates the wound,
My soft bandage relieves the sick.[4]

The *asû* was both a pharmacist and a prescriber of drugs, employing also a wide variety of empirical methods, such as lotions, suppositories, cataplasms, and enemas, and often relying for help on medical texts inscribed on cuneiform tablets. Whether the Mesopotamian who became ill initially sought assistance from the *āšipu* or the *asû* probably depended on whether the ailment was one for which a natural cause was readily apparent, in which case a person might well consult the *asû* directly. Undoubtedly some went first to the *āšipu* and then to the *asû*, either at the recommendation of the former or because he refused to treat the case. Some texts refer to both the *āšipu* and the *asû* working together on the same patient. But the *āšipu* used magico-religious methods of treatment, while the *asû* used natural methods. Occasionally, the same person would fill both roles, serving sometimes as an *āšipu* and sometimes as an *asû*.

We have seals belonging to physicians that reveal the existence of the *asû* in Sumer as early as 3000 BC, hence going back to the beginning of recorded history. Medical documents from Mesopotamia are numerous. Of the well over one hundred thousand cuneiform tablets that have been discovered, about eight hundred deal with medicine. The earliest medical text dates from the third dynasty of Ur (c. 2100 BC) and is written in Sumerian cuneiform. It contains fifteen prescriptions, of which eight are for poultices and three are for mixing medicines for internal consumption. Some cuneiform tablets contain a short description of a disease, its diagnosis, and a prescription of drugs and spells for treatment. The following is illustrative:

> If a man's tongue is swollen so that it fills his mouth, you dry tamarisk leaves, leaves of the *adaru*-plant, leaves of "fox-grape," [and] "dog's-tongue"-plant; you chop them up finely and sift; you knead them with juice of the *kasû*-plant; you rub the top of his tongue with butter; you put [the medication] on his tongue, and he will get well.[5]

In some cases one can see the transformation of omens into symptoms, that is, of supernatural into natural entities. The medical tablets mention diseases of the liver, the eye, respiratory diseases, fever, and gonorrhea. A catheter was used in the treatment of urinary-tract diseases. Some of the pathological conditions that are accurately diagnosed are tuberculosis, night blindness, inflammation of the middle ear, kidney stones, stokes, and scabies. The cuneiform tablets show that an extensive list of drugs were used, including mandrake and opium. There is no mention of surgery in the texts. It is likely to have been rare, probably limited to wounds in battle and accidents, such as being gored by a bull. We have no record of circumcision being practiced in Mesopotamia.

When one's sin is made responsible for one's suffering, as it was in Mesopotamia, it is inevitable that the problem of the apparently unjust suffering of the righteous person will arise. Between c. 2000 and c. 1700 BC a poem entitled "Man and His God," but usually referred to as the "Babylonian Job," was composed in Mesopotamia. It is the first known attempt to deal with the problem of human suffering—similar to the biblical Book of Job. In this poem a man presents his case to his personal god. He is plagued by sickness and other forms of suffering, yet he is aware of no wrong on his part. Instead of blaspheming his god, he humbly goes to him with tears, glorifies him, and laments and wails before him until his personal god is moved to pity and the sufferer's tears are turned to joy. The Babylonian Job learns two lessons: (1) the gods' values cannot be measured by human standards; and (2) a person's only recourse is to trust and hope. In this poem we have an instance of a man seeking healing directly from his god. The method, personal prayer, seems to have been the most common religious—and perhaps the only strictly religious—recourse for the ill in Mesopotamia. Reliance upon such a petition exclusively may well have been a last resort for those who had already availed themselves of the skills of those professionals who were engaged in healing.

Egypt

Egyptian civilization emerged on the banks of the Nile River only slightly later than Mesopotamian civilization. Egypt was a prosperous country, owing to the annual inundation of the Nile, which made the floodplain some of the most productive farmland in the Middle East. Egypt was united as a kingdom about 3000 BC, perhaps when the first pharaoh, Aha, united Upper (southern) and Lower (northern) Egypt.[6] Pharaonic Egypt is divided into three "kingdom" periods, each of which is subdivided into dynasties that were devised by an Egyptian priest named Manetho about 250 BC. His chronology has remained standard, with some modifications, since he created it. Since the nineteenth century the whole of Egyptian history has been divided into four great periods: the Early Dynastic Period (dynasties 1 and 2), c. 3000–2686 BC; the Old Kingdom (dynasties 3–6), 2686–2160 BC; the Middle Kingdom (dynasties 11 and 12), c. 2055–c. 1650 BC; and the New Kingdom or Empire (dynasties 18–20), c. 1550–1069 BC. These periods represent eras of prosperity and central control exercised by a pharaoh who ruled over the entire country. The three kingdom periods are separated by eras known as the First (c. 2160–2055 BC) and Second (c. 1650–c. 1550 BC) Intermediate periods, between the Old and Middle Kingdoms and the Middle and New Kingdoms, respectively, when central authority broke down and political and civil anarchy ensued.

We know much more about the medical techniques practiced in Egypt than we do about those of Mesopotamia because of several medical texts preserved on papyri. The Egyptians created a writing system perhaps during the Naqada III/"Dynasty 0" period (c. 3200–3000 BC). It began as a pictographic system of hieroglyphs and was eventually simplified into a cursive system, *hieratic*, which was used for rapid writing. Unlike the Mesopotamians, who wrote on clay tablets, the Egyptians wrote on papyrus, a form of paper made from the stem of the papyrus plant, which grows along the banks of the Nile River. Because of Egypt's extremely dry climate, thousands of papyrus fragments have been preserved in the sands of Egypt. Among them are more than a dozen scrolls of medical writings dating from c. 2000 BC to c. 1350 BC. (Ancient treatises were written on scrolls, not in volumes with pages as they are today.) Most are simply collections of drug recipes, but two of the medical papyri are much more extensive.[7] The first is the Papyrus Ebers (named for a German professor, Georg Ebers [1837–1898]), a kind of medical textbook dating to about 1550 BC. It is a scroll twenty meters long that was sold to Ebers by an Arab who said that it had been found between the legs of a mummy. It is without a doubt the most outstanding Egyptian medical document that has been preserved. It contains selections of several medical specialties (internal, skin, women's, and eye diseases). The papyrus includes 876 prescriptions made up of more than 500 substances, including lead and copper salts and many vegetable and animal substances, as well as *Dreckapotheke* (urine and human and animal excrements). Many of the concoctions are exotic and fantastic. One cure for baldness consists of a mixture of extracts from a female vulva, a male penis, and a black lizard. And the papyrus recommends smearing peppermint on a woman's buttocks to speed up a difficult birth. It also contains many cosmetic recipes, since the Egyptians set great store by beauty.

The second well-known Egyptian medical papyrus is the Edwin Smith Papyrus, which is a fragment of a longer scroll that describes forty-eight cases that involve injuries of the head, neck, chest, or shoulder. The verso gives magic treatments for other conditions. It was discovered at Thebes in 1862 and named after the young American Egyptologist, perhaps the first American to learn ancient Egyptian, who purchased it. It was first published in 1930 by James Henry Breasted. The papyrus is 15.4 feet long, beautifully written in black and red ink on both sides, and preserves about five hundred lines of hieratic writing from right to left in horizontal lines. It has been dated to about 1600 BC but was probably copied from a document written two or three hundred years earlier. The cases are arranged according to a pattern used by medical writers until the end of the eighteenth century: It starts with the head and ends with the heel (*a capite ad calcem*). It includes three categories of treatment for the physician: "an ailment I will treat"; "an ailment I will fight with" (where the outcome is less certain); and "an ailment for which nothing is done." Case 10 provides a representative example:

> Instructions concerning a wound in the top of his eyebrow. If you examine a man having a wound in the top of his eyebrow, penetrating to the bone, you should palpate his wound [and] draw together for him his gash with stitching. You should say concerning him: "[One having] a wound in his eyebrow. An ailment which I will treat." Now after you have stitched it, [you should bind] fresh meat upon [it] the first day. If you find that the stitching of this wound is loose, you should treat it with grease and honey every day until he recovers.[8]

The Edwin Smith Papyrus displays a high level of clinical observation, but unfortunately it is incomplete and ends at the level of the thorax. It was apparently an introduction to a much longer work and may have been intended for the use of military physicians. Although it is a surgical papyrus, no use of the knife is mentioned. Nearly all surgery that it describes is "mini-surgery," for bites by crocodiles, for example. Actual surgery is recommended only for superficial swellings and limited to external procedures. Most likely the only surgical tool available was a copper or stone scalpel. But the papyrus does include treatment of stitches and splints. Surgeons in most societies up to the latter half of the nineteenth century limited themselves to treating wounds and setting bones. In this papyrus there is an interesting case in which the surgeon is advised not to be diverted by the mystery of the symptoms. Without reference to the supernatural cause, the papyrus states that he is to attempt to deal with the symptoms themselves and conquer the ailment. While this should not be considered a rejection of the validity of magico-religious practices, it suggests (and other sources confirm) that there was a greater emphasis on naturalistic treatment among the

Egyptians than we find in Mesopotamian medicine. While the Edwin Smith Papyrus is considered the most rational Egyptian medical text, it includes eight magical incantations.[9] The Egyptians believed that malign forces could be overcome by the spoken word, especially in combination with amulets or talismans. Both natural and supernatural treatments were regarded as necessary, and they were used together in therapy. The papyrus mentions for the first time a practice that was to become common among physicians in nearly all ancient societies: that the physician would not treat hopeless cases.

In Egypt people who became ill and wished to avail themselves of the services of priests could go to those of Thoth, the divine physician of the gods, or those of the goddess Isis or of a wide range of other gods who were concerned with healing, including the deified Imhotep. In Egyptian belief, as in virtually every polytheistic religion, certain gods gave protection against specific diseases and, more unusual, each limb of the body was connected with a certain god. The gruesome god Bes, for example, was often depicted on amulets to ward off harmful gods. Women wore hairpins or jewelry that depicted the hippopotamus goddesses Ipi and Taweret for protection. These deities, however, were not the main sources of healing. There were three different kinds of healers to whom a sick person might go. The first, the *wabw*, was the priest of Sekhmet, a goddess of healing. The role of the priests of Sekhmet is a matter of dispute. Some scholars maintain that they were surgeons, others that they were originally only mediators between the patients and Sekhmet, mediators who had gradually acquired empirical techniques, particularly the use of drugs, which they combined with their magico-religious practices. The second, the *sa.u*, was a sorcerer or exorcist who used primarily charms and incantations, addressing the disease directly since it was considered to be the agent. Sometimes the *sa.u* would employ drugs as part of the treatment. Drugs in Egypt had not only a pharmacological value but a magico-religious one as well. Some were widely used specifically because of their association with magic or religion.[10] Natural substances such as honey (which was the main component in more than 900 remedies), pomegranate juice, and water lilies were used for treatment, and opium was used as a sedative.

The third healer, the *swnw*, was a physician similar to the *asû* in Mesopotamia. He or she (we know of two individuals identified by the feminine form, *swnw.t*), though not a priest, worshiped a patron deity, Thoth.[11] Some scholars believe that physicians were trained in schools, called Houses of Life, which were attached to temples (we know of five), and probably remained priests all their lives. Medicine was a specialized form of scribal education in which traditional texts were studied or memorized. The *swnw* was a physician of lower status who was paid by the state and served with the army or on building sites. He mingled prayers or incantations with a drug or procedure to intensify the healing power of the remedy that he applied. If an ailment had a natural cause, one probably went to a physician; if it seemed more complicated or mysterious, one probably first sought a priest or exorcist. At times two or even all three of these professions—the *wabw*, the *swnw*, and the *sa.u*—would be combined in one person. There was no rivalry between the three roles. In Egypt and Mesopotamia the empirico-rational and the magico-religious approaches were equally valid. Magical, religious, and naturalistic medicine existed side by side, overlapped, and sometimes blended, yet they were different although complementary systems, all compatible with one another and within a cultural ethos into whose fabric a magical and religious consciousness was woven.

There was a strong element of religious treatment within Egyptian medicine at all periods. In the Papyrus Ebers every treatment has to be followed by prayers and incantations to the appropriate god (Ra, Isis, and Horus were the most popular). Hence Egyptian medicine was always a blend of religious, magical, and natural medicine, although it was especially in those cases in which naturalistic procedures were ineffective that priestly and magical procedures were employed. The earlier medical papyri mingle them, while after the New Kingdom period, which ended c. 1069 BC, medical papyri seem to have become more magical, perhaps reflecting the growing superstition of Egyptian religion, which is evident in other sources. We cannot be sure, however, that medical texts that featured natural medicine have not been lost and only the magical treatments preserved. Cleanliness and hygiene are strongly emphasized in the medical papyri. Probably no ancient or modern society has so strongly insisted on personal hygiene as did the Egyptians. Egyptian males frequently shaved their hair and wore only loincloths, and they were circumcised. But cleanliness was not related to health so much as it was a manifestation of the concept of religious purity. The Egyptians had no understanding of the concept of contagion, and public sanitation was primitive.[12]

Physicians emerged as men of importance very early in Egypt. Athothis, whom Manetho names as the second king of the First Dynasty, is said to have practiced medicine and to have written anatomical works. The most famous of Egyptian physicians was Imhotep, a semilegendary but apparently historical vizier to the pharaoh Djoser (c. 2650–2600 BC). Although a physician by training, he was also regarded as a philosopher, high priest, and architect. He is considered to have designed and built the first Egyptian pyramid, the famous step pyramid at Saqqara. Imhotep was later deified as the god Ptah. He was known for his wisdom, and his aid was sought for infertility and healing. In many ways he resembled another culture hero, Asclepius, the Greek god of healing. Many bronze statuettes of Imhotep have survived. He is usually portrayed as a learned man with a papyrus roll on his knee, which may contain either medical writings or architectural plans. We know the names of about 150 medical practitioners who are called *swnw*, 52 from the Old Kingdom. One doctor, Nesmenau, functioned as a kind of general director for all medical work, suggesting that there was some kind of organization of the medical profession during the Old Kingdom. The same period gave us the world's earliest depiction of a surgical operation, circumcision. This portrait is cut into a doorpost of a royal tomb at Memphis. Herodotus states that circumcision was first practiced by the Egyptians and that its purpose was hygienic, though some scholars believe that it had a religious function.[13]

Egyptian medicine was said by Herodotus to be highly specialized. In the court of the pharaoh, every organ or sickness had its own specialist. One pharaoh had one doctor for his left eye and another for his right eye. Another royal physician was known as the "keeper of the royal anus." This specialization may be less an indication of advanced medicine than a carryover from primitive medicine, in which each organ or limb had its own god and therefore its own treatment. In fact, it is more likely that most physicians were general practitioners. The titles may simply represent positions in the medical hierarchy of the palace, since court physicians in Egypt were highly honored and organized in a rigid hierarchy. Egyptian doctors were known throughout the ancient Near East as the best in the world, and they were much in demand in royal courts outside Egypt.

Egyptian physicians were characterized by a strict traditionalism; they were not permitted to use new methods before trying old ones. This is a characteristic of ancient medicine in general, which, as a craft, favored tried and-true methods over novel ones. As craftsmen, Egyptian physicians were practical in their approach. The medical papyri avoid theory and speculation in favor of common-sense approaches to healing. Healers knew little about human anatomy. And even Egyptian undertakers, who regularly embalmed bodies, apparently had little interest in learning about human anatomy or physiology. Physicians did not perform autopsies, because to do so would be to show disrespect to the body, a view that has been held in many societies, and they probably had no contact with undertakers, who formed a separate caste. Hence most of what is stated about anatomy in medical texts is based on supposition rather than on the examination of cadavers. Physicians' understanding of physiology was similarly unsophisticated. They believed that the heart was the origin of thought and that blood was produced by the liver and cooled by the brain. Their writings do not discuss the process of healing or the reasons for drugs' efficacy.[14]

Hebrew and Jewish Medicine

While often overlapping, the terms *Hebrews, Israelites,* and *Jews* all refer to the same national and religious group, but in successive historical periods. *Hebrews* refers to the descendants of Abraham before their settlement in Palestine either c. 1450 BC or c. 1280 BC (the date is disputed), following the Exodus. *Israelites* refers to them from the time of their conquest of Palestine and the creation of the united kingdom of Israel in c. 1050 BC. This kingdom ended with the Babylonian conquest of Jerusalem in 586 BC, when the exiled Israelites became the *Jews* of the Diaspora. The rebuilding of the Temple in Jerusalem in 515 BC by Jews who had returned, following a decree of the Persian king Darius permitting them to do so, marked the beginning of the Second Temple period in Israel under a Jewish restoration, which ended with the Roman destruction of Jerusalem in AD 70. The three terms are often used interchangeably and not always with historical exactness.

The basic difference between the world-view of the Hebrews and that of their ancient Near Eastern neighbors was one of religious outlook. Israel's religion was normatively but not consistently monotheistic. The Hebrews were often monolatrous, worshiping one God (Yahweh), while not denying the existence of other gods. Israel was impacted throughout much of its history by the influence of its neighbors, who were polytheistic and who focused on the worship of natural forces, particularly those associated with fertility. Polytheism included an animistic element in which rivers, mountains, and trees were given spiritual qualities. Hebrew theology, as defined in the Old Testament, held that there was only one God, Yahweh, who was not part of nature but above and outside it as a distinct and independent spirit, the transcendent creator and sustainer of the world. Although Satan existed as a personal spiritual force of evil, he was subordinate to Yahweh and posed no independent challenge to his authority. In contrast to polytheism, which imposed no absolute moral standards, the ethical beliefs of Israel were grounded in the nature of Yahweh, whose absolute sovereignty gave authority to his revelation to Israel, while his holiness provided the moral basis of Israel's laws. The law of Israel, the Torah, grew out of Yahweh's covenant with the Hebrews, by which they perceived themselves to be a chosen nation. As a requirement of maintaining the covenant, Israel was to reflect in both personal and national life the moral character of Yahweh. Both justice and compassion were essential to his nature and were manifested especially in his relationship with his covenant people. Compassion, or "loving kindness," is a theme often found in the Old Testament. It implies a beneficence that goes beyond ordinary human relations, based on sympathy toward others, especially those who are suffering or in need.[15]

Central to understanding the theological framework of Hebrew and Jewish medical and healing practices is the concept of the image of God. In the Genesis Creation narrative, Yahweh is depicted as having made man and woman in his image.[16] Endowed with rationality, self-consciousness, and volition, the human personality was represented in Hebrew thought as mirroring Yahweh's image. Persons are spiritual beings, created to have communion with God and to be morally responsible for their actions. The concept of the image of Yahweh had implications for the protection of human life, which the Hebrews believed to possess intrinsic value and hence to be sacred. This view stood in marked contrast to that of surrounding cultures (Canaanite, Egyptian, Mesopotamian/Babylonian), in which persons were granted rights (including the right to live) by their parents, clan, society, or government. Even humans with physical defects were said to bear God's image. Yahweh asks Moses, "Who gives speech to mortals? Who makes them mute or deaf, seeing or blind? Is it not I, the Lord?" (Exod. 4:11).

Because of the Hebrew view of humanity as possessing intrinsic worth, the Torah exhibits a greater humaneness than do other codes of the ancient Near East, such as the Code of Hammurabi. There are provisions that protect the rights of the blind and the deaf (e.g., Lev. 19:14). The Torah is characterized by a pronatal approach. The fetus was regarded as having been created by Yahweh and designed for a specific purpose.[17] The newborn child was regarded as fully human and deserving of the same protection as an adult. Infanticide, a common practice in the surrounding Canaanite culture, was expressly prohibited, and the exposure of newborn children was also condemned.[18] Castration, sometimes practiced by Canaanites for religious purposes, was also forbidden, and eunuchs were excluded from Hebrew religious life (Deut. 23:1).

The Hebrews, like their neighbors, conflated natural and divine causation. Many Hebrews believed that disease and injury were a consequence of sin, but that they also lay clearly within Yahweh's control. Good and evil alike came from the hand of God, who said, "I kill and I make alive; I wound and I heal" (Deut. 32:39). Disease, as a manifestation of his wrath against sin, could be seen on both an individual and a national level. Thus Moses's sister Miriam was smitten with leprosy for questioning Moses's special relationship with God (Num. 12:1–16). The child that Bathsheba bore to David became sick and died on his seventh day because of David's sins of murder and adultery (2 Sam. 12:15–18). When Elisha's servant Gehazi accepted a reward from Naaman for his having been healed by the prophet, Yahweh smote Gehazi and his descendants with leprosy (2 Kings 5:25–27). On a wider scale, when David sinned by holding a census that was contrary to God's will, he was given the choice between seven years of famine, three months of war, and three days' pestilence upon his land. He chose the latter, and the "Lord sent a pestilence on Israel . . . and seventy thousand of the people died" (2 Sam. 24:10–17, esp. v. 15).

The tendency to moralize sickness by rendering its victims sinners in need of repentance was a late development in Egyptian and Mesopotamian religion, but it came to be widely held in antiquity that the sick were suffering deservedly because their disease was the result of offending the gods. A sick person was not viewed compassionately as an innocent sufferer but was seen as the recipient of deserved punishment. One finds this attitude everywhere in the ancient Near East. It is the attitude of Bildad the Shuhite, one of Job's comforters, who warns Job that Yahweh acts justly. Job and his sons have sinned against him, but if he repents and remains upright in his behavior, Yahweh will make him prosper (Job 8:1–10). Bildad's attitude transcends cultural boundaries and can be found in many societies. So deeply rooted was this assumption that it hindered the establishment of any general charitable concern for the sick.

But the Hebrews viewed suffering in general and sickness in particular not as the vindictiveness of a hostile deity, who had to be propitiated by means of ritual or offerings,[19] but rather as a chastisement that was corrective of the sins of his people. The classic case is that of Job. Small comfort was provided by Job's friends amid the calamities that befell him, one of whom said, "How happy is the one whom God reproves; therefore do not despise the discipline of the Almighty. For he wounds, but he binds up; he strikes, but his hands heal" (Job 5:17–18). Such an appraisal, although in accord with Old Testament thought, becomes for Job merely a heartless cliché. Job typifies the righteous sufferer, who was sorely tried but in the end was vindicated in his righteousness by God. The Book of Job presents a theodicy that rejects the widespread view found in the literature of the ancient Near East that sickness and disease were punishment for sin. When Yahweh asks Job who he is to question his ways, Job acknowledges the mystery of God's sovereignty and recognizes his inscrutable ways and ultimate goodness.

The Old Testament asserts God's justice, goodness, and mercy even while he afflicts his chosen people.[20]

For the Hebrews, Yahweh was the only healer (Exod. 15:26; see also Deut. 32:39). The Old Testament's incidental references to disease are often related to its moral or spiritual causes rather than to its merely physical nature. But to say that it was Yahweh who healed did not thereby rule out some perception of natural factors as a cause of disease, even if those factors were undefined or poorly understood. When the Philistines captured the Ark from the Israelites, they suffered from an epidemic of painful tumors (1 Sam. 5:6–12). But while they recognized the disease as divine punishment, they also drew a connection with the rats that were plentiful in Ashdod and Gath, where the Ark rested. When they returned the Ark to the Israelites, they sent as votive offerings five golden images of tumors and five of rats (1 Sam. 6:2–5). The episode indicates that the Philistines could posit a causal relationship between rats and disease, while at the same time attributing the plague to the anger of Yahweh.

The early Hebrews, like the Romans, were unusual in apparently having no native medical tradition and hence no native physicians. Like the Romans, they had recourse to both folk remedies and empirical medicines, which treated only symptoms without any theoretical understanding of disease. The Old Testament contains incidental references to binders of wounds, knowledge of setting fractures, and the employment of therapeutic substances. It is inconceivable that at any time the Israelites lacked knowledge of the rudimentary treatment of wounds and uses of herbs for various ailments in which natural causality was evident. In the Book of Exodus we find the stipulation that if a person injures another in a quarrel and the injured party survives, the one who inflicted the injury is to be held financially liable "for the loss of time, and to arrange for full recovery."[21] The last clause indicates that the expense of medicines, and perhaps of the services of the person dispensing or applying them, was to be borne by the guilty party.

Although there were surely healers among the Hebrews, we have no evidence that any systematized therapeutics existed in early Israel. The Israelites appear to have had no native practitioners similar to those elsewhere in the ancient Near East, where magic, religion, and medical empiricism coexisted in a medical context. The nomadic origins of the Hebrews may in part account for this absence, but an equally likely reason is the Israelites' reluctance to employ the magical or pagan healing practices employed in neighboring cultures, such as those of Egypt and Mesopotamia, for fear of religious syncretism. There is little evidence, however, to support the view that they held generally negative views of physicians or medicine. It is likely that they sometimes, perhaps often, employed medical craftsmen from Egypt and the Fertile Crescent, just as Romans employed Greek physicians, but tried to avoid the use of pagan religious and magical methods in Israel,[22] though in practice they must often have been indistinguishable from some of their own. Palestine lay within the orbit of both Egyptian and Mesopotamian/Babylonian cultures, and it was impossible not to be influenced by them. But magic was prohibited in the Mosaic code. Those practicing divination (soothsayers, augurs, sorcerers, charmers, mediums, wizards, and necromancers), if discovered, were to be put to death. In spite of this prohibition, Hebrews sometimes adopted magical practices from the indigenous Canaanite population.[23]

Belief in divine agency did not preclude the employment of natural means of healing, which were known and applied. We have reference to folk practices, such as the use of mandrake to remove sexual barrenness, and the belief that an aged man could prolong his life by drawing heat from a maiden's body.[24] When Hezekiah, king of Judah, became dangerously ill, the prophet Isaiah came to him and informed him, "Thus says the Lord: Set your house in order, for you shall die; you shall not recover" (2 Kings 20:1). When Hezekiah wept and prayed to God for recovery, Isaiah returned and told Hezekiah that God would add fifteen years to his life. Isaiah then instructed some unspecified attendants to take a cake of figs (probably a poultice) and apply it to the boil (perhaps a carbuncle) "that he may recover."[25] The occasional appeal to prayer, repentance, and fasting for healing does not imply that the Israelites regarded them as typical means of healing,[26] any more than is the case in religious cultures today. The Hebrews believed that all healing came from God. This was the case whether a disease was cured supernaturally or by a physician. Not only the patient but also the physician had to depend on God. Those who treated disease were considered his helpers, and they concentrated on treating the symptoms rather than the causes of disease, which God alone could heal. There is no evidence that the Jews regularly sought supernatural healing or had prescribed rites for religious healing. The Israelites of the Old Testament period did not ordinarily regard demons as the cause of disease, as did the Babylonians. With the introduction of demonology in the period of Second Temple Judaism, after the return of the Jews to Palestine from Babylon beginning in 538 BC, some disease came to be attributed to demons, although the common view remained that disease was the result of natural means and could be treated. The Hebrews did not lack medical knowledge, although the Old Testament suggests that their understanding of the causes of disease remained rudimentary and that treatment was largely confined to empirical medicine or folk remedies.

Ritual Purity and Leprosy

The concept of purity/impurity, or holiness/defilement, is one that the Hebrews shared with many ancient peoples.[27] Ritual purity denoted faithfulness to cultic requirements. Hence it was often used in the Old Testament and other ancient Near Eastern literature to symbolize moral purity.[28] To have clean hands was, metaphorically speaking, to have a heart that was free from moral pollution (sin). Hence ceremonial washing was a common religious preparation for worship in many ancient societies. In the Torah, ritual defilement resulted from participation in the normal course of human life and the cycles of birth, death, sex, and disease, which were unavoidable. When a Hebrew contracted ritual defilement, it was necessary for that person to undergo ritual purification. While the details in the Torah are explicit, we do not know how widely the regulations regarding ritual purification were followed.

According to the Torah, ritual defilement could come about in four ways: by contact with a dead body; by means of the discharge of bodily fluids associated with reproduction, such as semen or menstrual flow; by eating unclean foods, such as pork; and by contracting leprosy. The biblical regulations for ritual purity, which are found in Leviticus 11–16, are often referred to as the Holiness Code or the Law of Purity. Taken together, the taboos symbolized the holiness of Yahweh, who could not be approached carelessly, but only after a cleansing of body and heart and by means of restrictions that he had imposed. They also erected barriers against pagan religious practices and the possibility of syncretism with local Canaanite and other polytheistic religions, with their fertility and mortuary cults.

The dietary laws are the best-known regulations of the Holiness Code. Hebrews were forbidden to eat animals that the Torah said were unclean. Among quadrupeds those animals that had a cloven hoof and chewed the cud were pure and therefore edible (Lev. 11:3–8). But dogs, cats, camels, hares, and pigs could not be eaten, nor could rodents and reptiles. A distinction was made, moreover, between fish with fins and scales, which could be eaten, and fish without scales and fins, such as lobsters, crabs, shrimp, and other shellfish, which were unclean (Lev. 11:9–12). It has been suggested that fish with fins and scales were free-swimming, while those without scales and fins were not and would therefore act as hosts to parasites, particularly in slow-flowing and muddy rivers like the Nile. William Foxwell Albright surmised that these laws dated from the time the Hebrews lived in Egypt, since the distinction is not generally valid in salt water.[29] Unclean birds included vultures, buzzards, falcons, ostriches, hawks, sea gulls, owls, and bats, most of which are carnivorous or live in swamps and marshes (Lev. 11:13–19). The Torah also prohibited eating animals' flesh, with its blood, or eating blood. All pure animals had to be properly slaughtered, and no animal that died naturally or was torn by beasts could be eaten. In addition, ritual defilement was attached to bodily emissions, especially to sexual discharges, which also rendered a person impure. A man who had an emission of semen was impure until the evening, as was anything his semen touched until it was washed. A woman was impure for seven days from the beginning of her menstrual cycle. A man who lay with her also became unclean for seven days (Lev. 15:1–33).

It has been maintained, by Albright and others, that Hebrew laws regarding impurity of foods, disease, and sexual fluids had their basis in an empirical understanding of hygiene. Whereas in ancient Near Eastern medicine, such as that of Egypt and Mesopotamia, disease was often attributed to demons, in Hebrew culture it ordinarily was not. Of course, the Hebrews knew nothing of the organisms that spread disease. But Albright argued that their regulations regarding unclean fish, fowl, and animals may have been the result of experience in recognizing that particular diseases were transmitted by certain kinds of living creatures. Thus trichinosis was carried by pigs, tularemia by hares, and various diseases by birds that eat carrion. Most scholars today reject that view, which dates at least as far back as the physician Moses Maimonides (1135–1204).[30] While it has been argued that the familiar Jewish aversion to eating pork may initially have had an empirical basis, no health risk is associated with most of the animals and fowl categorized in the Holiness Code as defiling. Arabs enjoy camel meat, which they regard as a delicacy, but the camel was a prohibited animal. Moreover, many plants that were available to the Hebrews had greater risks to health than did prohibited creatures, and some were poisonous, but they are not listed as defiling. "There is, in the end, no direct association between health and purity, or between disease and defilement."[31]

The structural anthropologist Mary Douglas has suggested that ancient taboos such as those enshrined in the Holiness Code were neither primitive nor irrational.[32] Following Emile Durkheim, Douglas believed that like the rituals of every society, they reflected its values. They drew boundaries around Hebrew society that defined sacred space and provided a coherent pattern of what was and was not permitted, particularly in reference to approaching Yahweh in the tabernacle/temple, which was where he resided among the Hebrews. For Jews as for other ancient peoples, there was a close connection between the ideas of ritual purity and consecration to their God. Although to be ritually impure was not sinful (i.e., it did not involve transgression of the moral law), it was related to holiness. To the Hebrews ritual impurity symbolized moral pollution (sin), which was offensive to Yahweh and needed to be atoned for. Purification symbolized sanctification or being declared holy (*qādôš*) (Deut. 14:2). Indeed, holiness is the rationale given for the dietary prohibitions in Leviticus 11 (see 11:44–45). Holiness was perfection and completeness; it represented life and Yahweh. Hence dietary laws reflect the completeness of a particular class of creatures. Impurity symbolized death and deterioration. Taboos were not an early form of public health and hygiene; they symbolized holiness by establishing a rigid code of moral and ritual conduct, which were necessary to maintain the covenantal relationship with Yahweh. "Israel's attainment of holiness is dependent on setting itself apart from the nations and the prohibited animal foods. The dietary system is thus a reflection and reinforcement of Israel's election."[33]

In spite of the religious symbolism in the Hebrew understanding of disease and suffering that is everywhere evident in the Old Testament, priests in Israel did not function as physicians or surgeons, much less as diviners or exorcists, as they did in Egypt or Mesopotamia. They were involved, however, in various procedures for purifying those who had incurred defilement by childbirth, leprosy, seminal discharge, menstruation, and contact with a cadaver (Lev. 12, 13, 15, 21). A ritually impure Hebrew had to be purified by bathing, by making a sacrificial offering, or by the lapse of time. A priest's involvement was a matter of interpreting the law rather than of medical expertise. The closest that the priests of Israel came to occupying a medical role occurred when they were faced with examining a person to determine whether that person had the disease called "leprosy."

Biblical leprosy, as described in both Old and New Testament narratives, appears to encompass a spectrum of lesions that is broader than the modern Hansen's disease.[34] The latter is caused by a specific microorganism, *Mycobacterium leprae*, whose symptoms are a thickening of the skin with patches of discoloration and loss of sensation owing to the deterioration of the peripheral nervous system. But the Hebrew word *za'arath* (Gk., *lepra*) described a scaly condition that affected not merely the skin but also clothing and the walls of a house and probably included psoriasis, ringworm, and various fungal conditions. It is likely that the term was used in the Old Testament to describe a variety of conditions that produced suppurating sores and ulcers, which in their most severe forms disfigured and crippled their victims. There is no evidence that Hansen's disease existed in the ancient Near East, yet in the ancient world leprosy was regarded as the most loathsome of all diseases. Given the detailed ritual for cleansing lepers who had been healed, however, it appears that some forms of the disease could be and were healed. The vagueness of the symptoms in our sources makes it difficult to differentiate the various diseases that were subsumed under the term.

The laws concerning biblical leprosy reflect Hebrew ideas of contagion and infection, including the practice of quarantine. In Israel, whenever a swelling, eruption, spot, boil, or itch appeared on a person, that person had to appear before a priest, who quarantined him or her and periodically examined the person thereafter. He had the garments of a leprous person burned, and the leper was ostracized from society and treated as an outcast. The leper was to wear torn clothes and let his or her hair hang loose, cover the upper lip, and cry, "Unclean, unclean," so that people would stay away. Hebrew priests were to examine the house of a leper to determine whether it was infected. If it was, they were to close up the house for seven days. A house that could not be cleansed was torn down and its materials carried outside the city to an unclean place. This practice of isolating lepers may have been reasonable if some forms of leprosy were more virulent and contagious in the ancient world than they are now.

Hellenistic Jewish Medicine

We have no clear evidence of professional physicians in Jewish society until the Hellenistic period (323–30 BC). After Alexander's conquest of the Near East, Jewish communities both inside and outside Palestine underwent rapid Hellenization. As a result they were exposed to the Greek theoretical understanding of disease, which they adopted as compatible with their religious traditions. Greek medicine had been sufficiently divorced from its pagan religious background to be adapted to a variety of belief systems, including Judaism, as a value-free approach to healing. The readiness of Hellenistic Jews to accept Greek medicine can be seen in the apocryphal Wisdom of Jesus ben Sira (commonly known as Ecclesiasticus), which was written in Hebrew in the early second century BC and later translated into Greek in Alexandria, where many Jews had settled, by the grandson of the author. Although the Old Testament has little if anything to say about good health as a discrete concept, ben Sira reveals the influence of Greek medicine in praising it ("There is no wealth better than health of body") and in urging his readers to take suitable measures to care for their health by avoiding certain enumerated sins, such as gluttony, that shortened life.[35] A discussion of the role of physicians follows in chapter 38:1–15, where in a well-known passage ben Sira urges his readers to honor the physician because God has appointed him to heal. He receives his wisdom directly from God, who also produces medicines from the earth for men to employ. Healing by physicians is fully compatible with prayer, according to ben Sira, because it is ultimately God who heals. But the physician seeks the help of God so that his diagnoses will be successful and his treatment will save lives.

There is nothing in what ben Sira says about physicians that is discordant with the earlier spirit of Hebrew thought regarding medicine or healing. God heals through the physician, who is his agent. Ben Sira enlarges upon earlier principles and attempts to resolve the tension that might be thought to exist between reliance upon God and the practice of using theoretical medicine acquired primarily from pagan sources. His advice on prophylaxis is also noteworthy. In preliterate societies and in the ancient Near East (including Israel) health was thought to be preserved by punctilious attention to divine commands, as nearly all disease was seen in terms of divine causality. While a limited cause-and-effect relationship along natural lines was undoubtedly recognized in certain medical conditions, it remained for the development of Greek medical theory to introduce into lay consciousness a broader recognition of natural causality that led to the adoption of preventive measures and treatment, which were a part of Greek medicine. We know of Jewish physicians who practiced medicine in Palestine during Jesus's time. The Talmud recommends that every community have a surgeon, while a temple physician was maintained to treat the temple priests for abdominal diseases, by which they were especially troubled. Jews seem to have had little difficulty appropriating Greek medicine as being compatible with their theology.[36]

Even though in the Old Testament Yahweh is represented as the only healer and his people are commanded to refrain from resorting to magical or pagan healing practices, the use of natural or medicinal means is not forbidden; it is even employed in cases of supernatural healing by prophets. On the whole, medical knowledge was probably limited to folk remedies, however, and it is likely that there were no systematized therapeutics, much less a distinct medical profession similar to that of the magico-religious-empirical practitioners elsewhere in the ancient Near East. Not until the Second Temple period and the influence of Greek culture do we have evidence of a Jewish medical profession.

Chapter Two

Greece

The earliest Greeks, known as the Mycenaeans, settled on the Greek mainland before 1900 BC. They spoke an Indo-European language, but their place of origin is unknown. They founded several dozen fortified sites that eventually came under the hegemony of Mycenae, the most powerful city in Greece. Mycenaean Greece was a feudal society that was literate in the sense that a scribal class kept records. It traded extensively with the eastern Mediterranean and created a luxurious and highly structured palace culture. But at the end of the thirteenth century, for reasons that are not clear, the palaces were destroyed, Mycenaean society collapsed, and Greece descended into its Dark Age, from which it did not begin to emerge until the ninth century BC. The gradual resumption of trade with the Near East brought an ensuing economic revival, the creation of city-states (*poleis*), some of them built on abandoned Mycenaean sites, the adoption of the Phoenician alphabet and its adaptation to the Greek language, and extensive colonization, which carried Greek civilization throughout the Mediterranean and up the coasts of the Black Sea. In the Archaic Age (c. 750–c. 500 BC) the Greeks produced one of the most creative civilizations in the history of the Western world. Classical Greece reached its acme in the fifth and fourth centuries BC, with creative achievements in art and architecture, literature and philosophy, politics and history. As the city-states flourished, so did material and intellectual culture. Among their greatest accomplishments were the creation of rational or speculative medical theory and a tradition of naturalistic medicine that is commonly associated with Hippocrates.

The kaleidoscopic nature of Greek religion precludes a summary description. It possessed no creed or dogma and hence had no concept of orthodoxy or heresy; it had no sacred scriptures and no religious figures who obtained universal authority. Paganism was a religion of cultic worship; one could believe as little or as much as one wanted, but piety was judged by participation in public ritual, such as sacrifice, processions, and oracles. Much religious activity was of a local nature, rooted in the Greek city-state and enjoying little influence beyond a city's boundaries. There were deities that gained widespread worship and religious institutions, such as the Delphic oracle, that commanded respect over a wide geographical area. But without formal creeds or theologians to systematize belief, there was much disparity, not merely of time and place but even within the same community. Greek religion can perhaps best be described as a centuries-long accumulation of religious beliefs, myths, rituals, and practices that contained many layers and inconsistencies. As polytheists, the Greeks were not exclusive in their attitudes toward foreign gods. They not only respected the deities of other peoples with whom they came in contact (and often identified with their gods) but even incorporated them into the Greek pantheon.

The Archaic Age

The Greeks of Homer's time (Homer flourished perhaps c. 750–c. 725 BC), like the peoples of the ancient Near East, believed that the gods played an active role in all aspects of life, including sickness and health. Like the peoples of the Near East, they looked for supernatural causation in disease. In every culture societies have attempted to account for suffering in general and sickness in particular. We term these attempts *theodicies*. In the ancient world the most common explanation for suffering was that misfortune was retributive. Whenever epidemic disease was believed to result from supernatural intervention in human affairs, it was viewed as evidence of divine displeasure with humans for having violated a taboo or offended or provoked a god by insulting his or her honor in a way that was sometimes discoverable and sometimes not. When the gods were angry, they sent plague, drought, famine, flood, defeat in battle, or some other calamity. Diseases sent by the gods could be neither avoided nor healed until the anger of the gods was appeased by sacrifice or purification. Retribution could and did affect individuals or entire communities, in the latter instance sometimes owing to the fault of a single person. Homer's *Iliad* provides a well-known example.[1] The epic begins by describing a plague that has afflicted the Greek forces besieging Troy. The Greeks attribute the calamity to Apollo, who has for nine days been aiming pestilence-carrying arrows at his victims, with the result that piles of corpses are being burnt. On the tenth day a seer is consulted to determine why the god is angry. Once he discovers the cause (Agamemnon's refusal to accept a ransom in exchange for his daughter), the Greeks propitiate Apollo and the plague ends. Throughout antiquity, devastating natural disasters, such as plague, stimulated not only popular religious fervor but also the tendency to look for scapegoats. Thus natural disasters evoked persecution of early Christians in late antiquity on the ground that toleration of these "atheists" had provoked the wrath of the gods.

Beginning with Hesiod, who, like Homer, probably lived in the eighth century BC, we find an attitude toward disease that is quite different from that of Homer. In Homer's *Iliad* and *Odyssey* disease is sent by a god or caused by a *daimon* (an inferior spiritual being between gods and men) or other divine being.[2] It comes from outside the individual, but it is not the result of possession by either a god or a *daimon*. After Homer, however, we see the development of ideas of possession and the need for ritual purification. These ideas are found in the worship of Apollo and the Olympian gods or in the cult of Dionysus. In the former, the Delphic oracle taught the necessity of purification for pollution; the worship of Dionysus introduced the belief that a worshiper could be possessed and manifest hysterical behavior, such as outbursts of ecstatic dancing, sexual license, and engaging in a sacrificial rite called the *omophagia*, which consisted in tearing a live animal to pieces and devouring it raw. Divine possession manifested itself in less sensational ways, such as prophetic, poetic, or musical inspiration. It was natural that the concept of possession should be extended to the etiology of disease.

According to Hesiod in his *Works and Days*, evil, toil, and disease did not exist in early times. They came into the world as *daimones*, who escaped from Pandora's box as punishment of the human race for Prometheus's seizure of fire. "But countless other miseries roam among mankind; for the earth is full of evils, and the sea is full; and some sicknesses come upon men by day, and others by night, of their own accord, bearing evils to mortals in silence, since the counselor Zeus took their voice away."[3] For Hesiod, *daimones* is difficult to define. The word can refer to any divine agency, but its meaning is often vague and imprecise. Some *daimones* were kindly, but others, such as those to whom disease was attributed, were harmful.

The ancient Greek saw divine causation everywhere. Some events he ascribed to specific named deities, Olympian or other; but in the case of many events the answer to the question "why has this happened to me?" was "A *daimon* has sent this." Popular belief might assign particular functions to some *daimones*—each human being might have his own—but an infinity of these unseen powers remained for causing good or harm in general. . . . The word well illustrates the tangle of supernatural causation within which the ancient Greek passed his life.[4]

The early Greeks also thought that disease was caused by *keres* and *alastores*. *Keres*, like *daimones*, were malignant invisible powers that caused illness, misery, and death. They were neither personifications nor abstractions, but concrete though vaguely defined supernatural powers. The *alastores* were also evil spirits, believed to bring vengeance for homicide.

Since they believed that possession by a god or other divine power caused illness, the early Greeks turned for healing to a group particularly suited to the healing of heaven-sent illness, *iatromanteis*, or shamans. The *iatromantis* was a common feature of archaic Greek society. He wandered from city to city employing magic and religious means to avert disease and pollution. The *iatromantis* used herbs, spells, charms, exorcism, and various methods of purification. The Cretan poet Epimenides was an *iatromantis*, summoned to Athens in the seventh century BC, when the Athenians were suffering from a plague, to purify the city from pollution (*miasma*) that had been incurred by a sacrilege committed when a magistrate killed several men who had sought asylum in a temple. The Greeks believed that certain acts could pollute a whole people or city. This view was very much a part of the widespread ancient belief that the gods might bring retribution upon a whole society for an offence committed by one person.

The Greeks viewed the community as an aggregate of citizens who were kinsmen in the widest sense and who might therefore share in the misfortune of one of its members by experiencing his or her guilt or punishment. Hence an entire city or army might be afflicted by plague or other natural disaster brought about by an offence that had produced corporate guilt. Pollution could be introduced by a variety of actions, even those that were unintentional and therefore lacked moral guilt, such as accidental homicide or exposure to cadavers. A polluted person must be exiled or shunned to avoid contamination, and the pollution that the entire city incurred could be removed only by purification. The Greeks' belief in pollution provided an explanation for a communitywide disaster, an explanation that was based on the observation that even unintentional actions could upset the moral order and hence bring about negative consequences for society as a whole.

Of course, a disease might be divinely caused for reasons other than pollution. The Greeks believed that the gods sent disease for a variety of reasons. In Homer it was retribution for an insult or offence against a particular god. In post-Homeric belief, because the Greeks sought to relate justice to theology, they expected Zeus to punish injustice. It was a natural inference, and one frequently made in many societies, ancient and modern, that prosperity was a sign of divine favor and that suffering and disaster were indications of the gods' displeasure. Evidence of divine displeasure was seen by writers like Herodotus as divine *nemesis* (retribution), which struck down people if they enjoyed too much success. According to this view, the gods were jealous of prosperity and good fortune, which produced *hubris*, or overweening pride, in humankind. Yet, as it was apparent that the righteous do not always prosper but sometimes suffer injustice, while the wicked avoid deserved punishment and even flourish, the idea arose that a person could be punished for the deeds of his or her ancestors. Punishment had to be meted out in this life, there being little expectation of reward or punishment in the Greek conception of an afterlife.

Alongside a religious explanation of disease and attempts to expiate an offence that had caused it through the mediation of an *iatromantis*, there was in Homeric times a secular approach to medicine, found in the practice of physicians. Physicians exist in the *Odyssey*, where they are called *demiourgoi*, "men who work for the people." They were itinerant members of a craft, as were seers, carpenters, and heralds. They were not shamans, but they treated wounds empirically, relying on skill, observation, and experience. Beginning in the sixth century BC we hear of physicians in Greece called *iatroi*, who were concentrated particularly in Asia Minor and the Greek colonies in Sicily and southern Italy. However, we know little about them between the time of Homer and that of Hippocrates. Presumably the skill of medicine, like any other craft in Greek society, was transmitted by apprenticeship. Near the end of the sixth century BC, medical "schools" developed in various places in the Greek world, including Croton, Rhodes, Cyrene, Cnidus, and Kos. They were not schools in the modern sense but guilds of physicians who attracted students to serve as apprentices under them.

Fifth-Century Medicine

It was in a medical center on the island of Kos, off the coast of Asia Minor, that the famed Hippocrates (c. 460–c. 380 BC) lived. In spite of his reputation as the "father of medicine," the embodiment of medical wisdom, and the exemplar of the ideal physician, we know little about Hippocrates's life. There are only a few contemporary or near-contemporary references to him. He is mentioned by Plato, Aristotle, and Aristotle's pupil Menon.[5] He is said to have been a native of the island of Kos and to have been an Asclepiad (the term may refer to a family or a guild of physicians that traced their origin to Asclepius, the god of healing, or it may simply mean "physician"). He was, according to these sources, a teacher of medicine whose fame Plato compared to that of the sculptors Polyclitus and Phidias. He taught that one could not understand the body without taking into account the whole, and he explained disease as the result of air that formed in the body during the process of digestion. A biographical tradition that began long after his lifetime incorporated additional details, many of them anecdotal and legendary. Four short biographies are extant. It is uncertain how much of the information they contain is trustworthy. They relate that Hippocrates learned medicine from his father, Heraclides, who was a physician; that he studied under the atomist Democritus and the sophist Gorgias; that he traveled extensively in Greece, visiting Athens, northern Greece, and the Propontis (the present-day Sea of Marmara); that he taught medical students on Kos; and that he died at an advanced age at Larissa, in Thessaly, where he was buried. Additional biographical material contained in a collection of spurious epistles attributed to Hippocrates is almost certainly fictitious.

Hippocrates probably first became the subject of widespread interest during Hellenistic times (323–30 BC), when a large and heterogeneous collection of anonymous medical works—the Hippocratic Corpus—was attributed to him. They number some sixty treatises, all written in the Ionic dialect. Most of them date from the late fifth or fourth century BC, but some are much later. The collection, which may have originated as the library of a medical school, perhaps that of Kos, was brought to Alexandria in the third century BC, where it came to be attributed to Hippocrates. All the works are anonymous, and they exhibit differences of style and approach. It is widely held today that none can be attributed with certainty to Hippocrates. It is possible that he wrote some of them, but there is no agreement on which, if any, are authentic, and many historians of medicine doubt that any were authored by him. Some were written by physicians and are of a clinical nature, while others were composed by lay writers to appeal to an interest in medicine and medical theory among the general public. Still others were composed by professional teachers of philosophy or rhetoric and are more theoretical. To speak of "Hippocratic medicine" is to refer to views that are set forth in treatises that traditionally have been attributed to Hippocrates.

The deontological treatises of the Hippocratic collection (treatises that address moral obligation) are the earliest writings that deal with medical etiquette and professional ethics. They seek for the first time to create a distinct identity for the physician and to lay down guidelines for professional conduct. In establishing a standard of behavior by defining the obligations of the physician, they created both a tradition of medical ethics and an ideal of dedicated practice, which were subsequently adopted in late antiquity and the Middle Ages. They have continued to influence the Western medical tradition to the present day, and they remain the greatest legacy of Hippocratic medicine. The best-known of the Hippocratic treatises is the so-called Hippocratic Oath:

> I swear by Apollo Physician and Asclepius and Hygieia and Panaceia and all the gods and goddesses, making them my witnesses, that I will fulfill according to my ability and judgment this oath and this covenant:
>
> To hold him who has taught me this art as equal to my parents and to live my life in partnership with him, and if he is in need of money to give him a share of mine, and to regard his offspring as equal to my brothers in male lineage and to teach them this art—if they desire to learn it—without fee and covenant; to give a share of precepts and oral instruction and all the other learning to my sons and to the sons of him who has instructed me and to pupils who have signed the covenant and have taken an oath according to the medical law, but to no one else.
>
> I will apply dietetic measures for the benefit of the sick according to my ability and judgment; I will keep them from harm and injustice.
>
> I will neither give a deadly drug to anybody if asked for it, nor will I make a suggestion to this effect. Similarly I will not give to a woman an abortive remedy. In purity and holiness I will guard my life and my art.
>
> I will not use the knife, not even on sufferers from stone, but will withdraw in favor of such men as are engaged in this work.
>
> Whatever houses I may visit, I will come for the benefit of the sick, remaining free of all intentional injustice, of all mischief and in particular of sexual relations with both female and male persons, be they free or slaves.

What I may see or hear in the course of the treatment or even outside of the treatment in regard to the life of men, which on no account one must spread abroad, I will keep to myself holding such things shameful to be spoken about.

If I fulfill this oath and do not violate it, may it be granted to me to enjoy life and art, being honored with fame among all men for all time to come; if I transgress it and swear falsely, may the opposite of all this be my lot.[6]

Precisely when the oath was written is uncertain. Although its earliest mention is by Scribonius Largus in the first century AD, it may date from as early as the fourth century BC. There is no evidence of its use for admission to the practice of medicine in the pre-Christian era. In Greece a physician was a person who claimed to be a physician, and no oath was required of him. Those who took the Hippocratic Oath swore by Apollo, Asclepius, and other gods and goddesses of healing to guard their life and art "in purity and holiness." Its religious tenor and some of its injunctions suggest that it originated among a restricted group of physicians. It differs in several particulars from the mainstream of Greek medical ethics, which did not prohibit abortion, euthanasia, or surgery. It was regarded by some pagan medical writers during the Roman imperial period as setting forth an ideal standard of professional behavior, but at no time was it used in the classical world to regulate the practice of more than a minority of physicians. The oath was later adopted by Christians, Jews, and Muslims, and with necessary changes it gained wide use, but how extensively it was known in the classical period is not clear.

It was in the fifth century BC that Greek medicine began to take on the form of a science as well as that of a craft. A science requires the existence of a body of theoretical knowledge, which can hardly be said to have existed in medicine before the late fifth century BC. There were, of course, many empirical techniques that had been collected and transmitted, but they could not be called a body of knowledge. The medical practitioner could identify symptoms and supply details about illnesses, and he (we do not know of any female physicians at this time) might be skilled at treatment, which consisted in applying traditional remedies, but there was no attempt to understand disease in broad terms or to frame general theories that could be applied to particular cases. It was the addition of the theoretical aspects of medicine and disease that led to the creation of "scientific" or "rational" medicine in antiquity. Such medicine, which tried to explain disease in terms of natural causation, was beyond the skill and competence of the ordinary practitioner. Those physicians who attempted a more theoretical understanding of disease and its etiology turned to philosophy, which they believed could provide a correct understanding of human nature and furnish universal formulations. Philosophers constructed physiological theories by which physicians could explain illness and provide treatment. Physiology did double duty as a branch of both natural philosophy, which dealt with the natural sciences, and medicine. In both subject areas physicians and philosophers read the same medical treatises and debated the same topics. As part of natural philosophy, physiology became a component of the general education in the schools of the ancient and medieval worlds, and educated laymen often displayed a detailed knowledge of physiological theory. In early Christian times the subject was incorporated into theological works, particularly of apologetics, and was widely discussed by Scholastic theologians in the High Middle Ages.

In the Hippocratic Corpus we see the earliest attempts to provide a theoretical basis for the practice of medicine. Most Hippocratic treatises reveal an approach to medicine that is both rational and empirical: rational in its freedom from belief in divine etiologies and in its search for natural causes of disease, empirical in the collection of case histories that give careful descriptions of symptoms based on meticulous clinical observation. Their case histories remained unparalleled until the sixteenth century. Regarding health as the natural state, Hippocratic physicians recognized the healing force of nature (*vis medicatrix naturae*) and attempted to assist the body to heal itself. They borrowed materialist theories of the nature of health and disease from the physiological speculations of the pre-Socratic philosophers, who attempted to explain the world in terms of natural processes rather than in terms of mythological categories.

Perhaps the best-known theory was based on the system of quaternaries, the four humors derived from Empedocles,[7] according to whom the body contained four fluids (blood, phlegm, yellow bile, and black bile), which were analogous to the four elements of matter (air, water, fire, and earth) and which produced four qualities (warmth, cold, wetness, and dryness). Many doctors believed that health resulted from a harmonious blending (*krasis*) of the humors of the body, while disease was caused by a disturbance or imbalance of humors. That balance was created by employing the six "non-naturals" (air, diet, exercise and rest, sleep and waking, evacuation and retention, and passions of the mind), which could tip the body into either disease or health. Treatment consisted in creating an individual regimen of hot or cold foods that would counterbalance the disease with a contrary, together with drugs and cautery or bloodletting.

The fact that the body's secretion of various fluids, such as vomit, feces, urine, and nasal discharge, is often a symptom of the physiological change that accompanies sickness probably accounts for Greeks' attention to what they would call "humors." According to the theory that was given its final formulation by Galen in the second century AD, all four humors were found in the blood and were capable of being transformed into a noxious humor or superfluity, which had to be drawn, usually from a vein in the arm, in order to heal the patient by restoring nature's proper balance. Phlebotomy was believed to do this, and its use became popular, even more so than cautery, which was painful and therefore avoided when possible. Knowledge of the human body was limited largely to surface observation, with the study of anatomy, physiology, and pathology playing little part in medicine until the Hellenistic period. Hence surgery was confined to the body's surface.

The Greeks also ascribed psychological temperament to a material cause, an excess of one or another humor, with the excess of each producing an associated temperament (sanguine, phlegmatic, choleric, or melancholic). The cause for each temperament of the human personality was a specific bodily fluid or humor, not a psychological factor. Traces of the older, prerational mentality can be found in some of the Hippocratic treatises that are not wholly free from pretheoretical concepts of disease. But in general they reveal a wedding of speculative philosophy with medicine, which provided the theoretical underpinning that made Greek medicine fully naturalistic in its approach by the late fifth century BC. Treatment by physicians usually consisted of one of three types of therapy, in order of preference: diet, drugs, or surgery.

This approach to medicine is seen in an interesting Hippocratic treatise, *The Sacred Disease*. Madness was often popularly regarded as a punishment by the gods. Thus Herodotus wrote that the madness that afflicted the Persian king Cambyses was explained as the result of his offending the Egyptian god Apis.[8] Epilepsy was similarly thought to be caused by divine possession, a view that is rejected by the author of *The Sacred Disease*. He begins by stating, "I am about to discuss the disease called 'sacred.' It is not, in my opinion, any more divine or more sacred than other diseases, but has a natural cause, and its supposed divine origin is due to men's inexperience, and to their wonder at its peculiar character." He sharply distinguishes his rational outlook from the traditional view:

> My own view is that those who first attributed a sacred character to this malady were like the magicians, purifiers, charlatans and quacks of our own day, men who claim great piety and superior knowledge. Being at a loss, and having no

treatment which would help, they concealed and sheltered themselves behind superstition and called the illness sacred, in order that their utter ignorance might not be manifest.

Near the end of the work he writes, "There is no need to put the disease in a special class and to consider it more divine than the others; they are all divine and all human. Each has a nature and power of its own; none is hopeless or incapable of treatment."[9]

The theology underlying the statement that all diseases are both sacred and human does not reflect popular opinion, according to which certain diseases, such as epilepsy, were caused by particular gods or divine forces. Rather it is derived from the pre-Socratic philosophers. This view rejects the direct interference of the gods in the natural order but regards every natural event as divine. The physician was freed by this view to seek natural causes of disease. Hence, the author of *The Sacred Disease* can explain epilepsy as being due to "the things that come and go from the body, from cold, sun, and from the changing restlessness of winds." This natural explanation of disease became one of the hallmarks of the Hippocratic physician, though it did not indicate a merely mechanical understanding of nature.

How did Greek laymen of the classical period react to this naturalistic approach to disease? Did they retain a supernatural etiology of disease? With the growth of rationalism in the latter half of the fifth century BC and the widespread influence of the sophistic movement, which popularized relativistic views throughout Greece by means of itinerant lecturers (sophists), who created what has been termed the fifth-century Enlightenment, naturalistic explanations displaced traditional supernatural views for many, especially among the younger generation, who enthusiastically accepted the views of the sophists. A significant lay interest in medical questions developed, with the result that a number of Hippocratic treatises were addressed to a general audience. They must have done much to spread the new views of medicine. And it is likely that those who sought help from Hippocratic physicians expected them to be guided by treatment based on physicians' theoretical principles.

Was there a conflict between traditional religion and the new emphases of Hippocratic medicine? Since the time of Homer, physicians had been a feature of Greek life. Even in the Archaic Period, when plague and disease were widely thought to be the result of divine punishment or *daimones*, empirical medicine was recognized as a legitimate approach to illness, the treatment of wounds, and the setting of fractures and dislocations. It was much less efficacious for epidemic diseases, however, for which medicine could do little and which the Greeks still attributed to the anger of the gods.[10]

There is no reason to assume that in the fifth century BC, when theoretical medicine predominated, secular medicine was viewed with suspicion. Since Hippocratic writers did not deny the divinity of nature, they did not offend popular belief. When they described disease as the result of natural processes, they were not excluding recognition of divinity, for nature itself was regarded as divine. Their theology was naturalistic but not atheistic. Medicine was recognized as a divine art that had been given to humanity by a god. It was trusted and looked to for aid. "I have discovered regimen, with the god's help, as far as it is possible for mere man to discover it," concludes the author of *Regimen*. The Hippocratic attitude toward religion was not hostile. "In fact, it is especially knowledge of the gods that by medicine is woven into the stuff of the mind," according to the author of *Decorum*. "Physicians have given place to the gods, for in medicine that which is powerful is not in excess. In fact, though physicians take many things in hand, many diseases are also overcome for them spontaneously. . . . The gods are the real physicians, though people do not think so." Prayer was not rejected. In *Regimen* we read, "Prayer indeed is good, but while calling on the gods a man should himself lend a hand."[11] However, there is little advice in the Hippocratic Corpus for the physician or patient to resort to prayer alone for the healing of disease. The reason is not hostility to religion but rather the belief that prayer should be used to thank the gods rather than to ask them for favors.

The Plague of Athens

Epidemic diseases did not fit easily into the framework of Greek medical theory or of traditional theodicies. This became apparent during the great Plague of Athens, which struck Athens in the early summer of 430 BC and continued during the following year, with several recurrences, the first in 427 BC. The plague was the first major epidemic described in human history and the best-known of several in the classical world thanks to the classic description by Thucydides,[12] which influenced both subsequent plague descriptions and the perception of epidemic disease itself. The dramatic force of the narrative brings out all the characteristics of many of the major plagues in history: the virulence of an epidemic disease when it attacks a society that has not previously been exposed to it, the high mortality rate, and the social and moral dislocations that it often produces in the society that experiences it.

The plague is an example of a new epidemic that beset a population previously unacquainted with the disease. The conditions of the Athenians could not have been worse. A population of as many as 350,000 men, women, and children who had previously lived in a dozen villages scattered across Attica were packed into the narrow space inside the city walls (about three square miles) during the second summer of the Peloponnesian War (431–404 BC), while Athenian territory was under siege by the Spartans. Food was scarce, conditions were crowded, with many living in poorly ventilated shacks or tents in hot summer, hygiene was poor, and the contagious disease spread quickly. Outside the walls the Spartans laid waste to the Athenians' territory, poisoned their wells, and cut down their olive trees, which for almost two centuries had provided the greatest agricultural resource of Athens.

It has been suggested that Thucydides's account of the plague, which he had himself contracted, was influenced by Hippocratic medicine and particularly by Hippocratic writers' careful descriptions of the course of the disease. Thucydides believed that the plague, which began in Ethiopia, had been brought to the Athenian port of Piraeus by grain-bearing ships from Egypt and Libya. From Piraeus it spread within the walls into the city of Athens itself. Thucydides recorded the symptoms in detail, hoping that future generations would be able to recognize the epidemic if it should reappear. They included severe headaches, bleeding from the mouth and throat, and inflamed eyes, followed by respiratory symptoms such as sneezing, coughing, and chest pains. In a third stage the illness affected the gastro-intestinal tract, producing stomach cramps, vomiting, and diarrhea, which were accompanied by unquenchable thirst. Other symptoms were rash, blisters, gangrene, amnesia, and delirium. Death often occurred on the seventh, eighth, or ninth day, though survivors of the first stage sometimes died from the effects of diarrhea. Those who survived gained some immunity, since if they contracted the disease again it did not prove fatal, but they sometimes lost their memory, sight, or, because of gangrene, the use of their extremities. The plague carried off between one-quarter and one-third of the entire population of Athens, perhaps between 75,000 and 100,000 people, including the Athenian statesman Pericles, who died in 429 BC.

Given Thucydides's detailed account of the plague, it is ironic that we cannot identify the specific disease or diseases that were responsible for it. More than thirty suggestions have been made regarding its identity, including measles, smallpox, typhus, ergotism, and scarlet fever. Epidemic smallpox and typhus are the most often suggested. Every few years someone postulates a new theory. In

1985, for example, scholars suggested that the Athenian plague was a combination of influenza and toxic shock syndrome, though the latter had been diagnosed for the first time in 1978. A more recent theory identified it as Rift Valley Fever. These suggestions, like nearly all others, have convinced few scholars, and it is likely that the disease entities no longer exist. DNA examination of skeletal material from a mass burial pit of 160 corpses discovered in 1994–95 in the Athenian Kerameikos, a cemetery that dates roughly from the time of the plague (c. 430 BC), has not made possible a certain identification of the disease, though typhoid fever has been suggested.[13]

What is most striking about Thucydides's narrative is his description of the mass psychology that characterized the plague victims. The disease brought about a complete breakdown of societal norms and traditional morality. Many Athenians who saw their relatives and friends succumbing to the plague became convinced that they would soon die themselves. They prayed to the gods for help, but when the disease continued unabated, they began to think that their prayers and offerings made no difference. As a result, the traditional restraints of morality and law broke down. Demoralized Athenians turned to pleasure-seeking, lawlessness, and extravagant and erratic behavior. Ecstatic and orgiastic rites spread throughout the population, while traditional burial rites, which had played an important role in Greek religious piety, were ignored.

> Terrible, too, was the sight of people dying like sheep through having caught the disease as a result of nursing others. This indeed caused more deaths than anything else. For when people were afraid to visit the sick, then they died with no one to look after them; indeed, there were many houses in which all the inhabitants perished through lack of any attention. . . . The bodies of the dying were heaped one on top of the other, and half-dead creatures could be seen staggering about in the streets or flocking around the fountains in their desire for water. The temples in which they took up their quarters were full of the dead bodies of people who had died inside them.[14]

The Athenians, finding that the traditional gods had failed to help them, sought the aid of new deities. The most prominent was Asclepius, whose worship was introduced in Athens in 420 BC, with several prominent Athenian citizens, such as the playwright Sophocles, leading the initiative to introduce his cult. The gods' failure to intervene to prevent or stop the plague did much to undercut traditional religion in Athens and to prepare the way for the skeptical teachings of the sophists in the late fifth century BC.

The Cult of Asclepius

In addition to the development of theoretical medicine in Greece during the fifth century BC, there was a tradition of religious healing in which patients sought a cure directly from a god rather than from a physician. Those people who sought divine help for healing could appeal to a wide variety of gods, demigods, and heroes. Originally there were no special gods of healing, and any deity could be invoked by the sick. Many local cults of healing grew up around holy sites that were regarded as the burial places of heroes, mighty men, real or mythical, who were thought to give aid in time of need and who might be appealed to for healing.

Perhaps beginning as one such hero, Asclepius came to be the chief healing god of Greco-Roman antiquity. Asclepius is mentioned in the *Iliad* as a mortal, the "blameless physician," who was taught medicine by Chiron. Hesiod and Pindar speak of him as a son of Apollo and Coronis and say that he became famous as a physician and even restored the dead to life, for which he was slain by a thunderbolt of Zeus. Later legend made him a god. His cult seems to have originated at Tricca, in Thessaly, in northern Greece, but it spread to Epidaurus, in the Peloponnese, perhaps in the sixth century BC, and it was there that it first attained real prominence. The cult later spread throughout the Greek world: to Athens in 420 BC, to Pergamum in Asia Minor and to Kos, both in the fourth century BC, to Lebena in Crete, to Cyrene in North Africa, and in 291 BC to Rome, where the god was worshiped under the Latin name Aesculapius. The dissemination of his cult often followed an epidemic disease, as did his arrival in Athens and Rome. Asclepius gradually attracted to himself the healing functions of many of the other Greek gods and heroes. Perhaps he owed his success as the healing god par excellence to his association with Apollo and the support of the Delphic oracle or to the zeal of the priests at Epidaurus in promoting his cult.

It is noteworthy that the rapid spread of the cult of Asclepius began in the fourth century BC, when there was a marked decline in the traditional civic religions and an increase in the number of cults that offered the personal spiritual comfort that had been lacking in the civic cults. It was also the age that saw the spread of the Hippocratic type of medicine. The worship of Asclepius appealed to the rising individualism in Greece that characterized the century, and it evoked a personal devotion to the god that was not often found in the formal civic religions, particularly those of the Olympian gods.

There was in Greece from early times a group of physicians, called Asclepiads, who claimed descent from Asclepius; they were found at Kos and at Knidos in Asia Minor, among other places. Since one of the three Panhellenic healing sanctuaries of Asclepius was on the island of Kos, off the coast of Asia Minor, the alleged birthplace of Hippocrates, it used to be believed that Hippocratic medicine grew out of the healing associated with the temple of Asclepius and that the Asclepiads were priest-physicians. A tradition in antiquity was that Hippocrates came to understand the importance of gathering clinical cases and employing dietetics from accounts of cures posted in the temple at Kos. Theoretical medicine in Greece was thought to have its origins in the religious medicine practiced by the priests of Asclepius. This theory has been shown to be untenable by archaeological excavations at Kos, which revealed that the sanctuary of Asclepius was not founded until the fourth century BC, after the age of the origin of Hippocratic medicine, and therefore cannot have been the cradle of Greek theoretical medicine. But the later connection of the two approaches is noteworthy.

Emma and Ludwig Edelstein, in their definitive study of Asclepius, have suggested that Asclepius began as a culture hero and became the patron of physicians who practiced their art as wandering craftsmen. The name *Asclepiads*, meaning "sons of Asclepius," came to be adopted by those who practiced medicine and considered themselves descendants of the hero. He gave them the protection that they needed as itinerant physicians and was a god to worship who was not tied to a particular place. The Asclepiads were never priest-physicians. Eventually Asclepius's reputation was spread by physicians, until he became the chief healing god, and over time he eclipsed all others. He was deified perhaps at the end of the sixth century BC. In the fifth century his cult began to spread from Epidaurus to the rest of Greece, and in the fourth century it reached Kos, where the Koan physicians adopted him as their patron. Once sanctuaries of Asclepius were established in Kos and elsewhere, Hippocratic medicine and temple healing flourished side by side. The cult spread throughout the Mediterranean world until there were several hundred temples and shrines dedicated to Asclepius, either alone or with other gods.

As the chief healing god of Greece, Asclepius was sought out by the sick, who visited his temples seeking miraculous healing, often for diseases that physicians could not cure. They came from all over the Mediterranean world, though each of the three main sanctuaries attracted pilgrims especially from nearby cities. When pilgrims arrived, they first had to undergo a rite of bathing for purification, for ritual purity was required of those who wished to approach the god. Over the entrance to the temple at Epidaurus were the words, "Pure must be he who enters the fragrant temple; purity means to think nothing but holy thoughts." The pilgrim offered sacrifices (usually cakes and fruits and sometimes a pig) and could read testimonials (*iamata*) written on marble tablets in the sanctuary that told of instances of miraculous healing. Excavation has brought to light three such tablets at Epidaurus dating from the fourth century BC. They relate some seventy case histories of alleged miraculous cures, such as that of Gorgias of Heracleia:

> Gorgias of Heracleia with pus. In a battle he had been wounded by an arrow in the lung and for a year and a half had suppurated so badly that he filled sixty-seven basins with pus. While sleeping in the Temple he saw a vision. It seemed to him the god extracted the arrow point from his lung. When day came he walked out well, holding the point of the arrow in his hands.[15]

The tablets were doubtless intended to encourage the faithful to trust the god for healing. The actual process of healing involved incubation, the practice of having pilgrims spend the night in the *abaton*, the holiest part of the temple, where they were to lie on a couch and wait for a dream or vision of the god in which Asclepius would appear to heal them or to advise them regarding which therapy to follow. Sometimes the suggested therapy was dietary, and sometimes it involved recipes for ointments or other kinds of external treatment. The Greeks probably borrowed the practice of sleeping in a temple to obtain healing from Egypt, where it apparently extended back to the New Kingdom. The god often appeared holding a staff with a snake coiled around it, the caduceus, which became associated with him and remains an icon of the medical profession today. Sometimes he merely touched incubants (those who slept in the *abaton*), sometimes he operated on them or administered medicine, and sometimes a sacred serpent or dog would lick their wounds. When incubants awoke the next morning, they might find themselves cured. Votive offerings testifying to actual cures have been found in considerable numbers at the sanctuaries of Asclepius. The most interesting are terra-cotta models of eyes, ears, limbs, and other organs that Asclepius healed.

What kinds of disease were cured by Asclepius? Pilgrims sought healing for a wide variety of ailments—infertility, blindness, dropsy, paralyzed limbs, kidney stones. Henry Sigerist suggests that many pilgrims probably suffered either from chronic diseases or from psychogenic illnesses.[16] The latter are known to respond well to faith healing, but the cure is usually not permanent. In this regard the "miraculous" healings furnish evidence of ancient psychotherapy. But the healing offered by Asclepius probably represented a last hope for those whose diseases could not be, or had not been, cured by physicians. Women who were childless sometimes sought help. Several cases recorded on the marble tablets are clearly fictional, such as that of the woman who gave birth to a child she had carried for five years, or that of the woman who received a new eye in her vacant eye socket. The incubants sometimes dreamed of operations or the administration of medicine by Asclepius, who seemed to heal as a physician might be expected to, that is, by ordinary medical means.

Eventually around the temple of Asclepius at Epidaurus and elsewhere buildings were constructed to adorn the sanctuary and entertain pilgrims, such as theaters, stadiums, gymnasiums, sanatoriums, and baths. There were guesthouses for patients who required a long stay. The athletic facilities were used for the celebration of the festival of Asclepius.

One might expect to find an antagonism between secular and religious medicine as represented on the one hand by physicians and on the other by the numerous sanctuaries of Asclepius. Yet such antagonism seems to have been lacking in the classical world. Asclepius was the patron of both physicians and patients. He presided over the practice of secular medicine. Physicians who took the so-called Hippocratic Oath, if indeed any did, swore by Asclepius and other healing gods. In Athens, physicians sacrificed to Asclepius and Hygieia (the personification of Health, who was the daughter of Asclepius) twice each year for themselves and their patients. The celebrated physician Galen (AD 129–c. 217) called himself a servant of Asclepius, "since he saved me when I had the deadly condition of an abscess."[17]

Physicians generally accepted the validity of divine dreams and had no philosophical objections to religious healing. Rather, religious medicine was viewed by physicians as complementing their own practice. When Greek physicians believed they could no longer help a patient, they refused to give further treatment. The patient was regarded as beyond the point at which natural medicine could help, and so physicians freed the patient to seek other means, including the direct help of the god Asclepius. Physicians were not jealous of the god's ability to heal in cases where they could not, particularly in cases of chronic disease, which physicians were reluctant to treat because they could do so little. Hence one cannot speak of a conflict between religious and secular medicine, for both were aspects of healing that came from the same god. On Kos, physicians were situated side by side with the temple of Asclepius, which formed a leading center of healing in the Greek world. While the two healing traditions were separate from one another, they apparently enjoyed mutual respect.

During the Hellenistic period, following the death of Alexander the Great in 323 BC, a number of foreign deities, such as Isis and Serapis from Egypt and Mithra from Persia, came into Greece from the Eastern world. They were brought back to Greece by soldiers who had served with Alexander and his successors on campaigns in the East. The Hellenistic period was a cosmopolitan age, and the Greeks' frequent travel and resettlement facilitated the rapid spread of these cults throughout the Mediterranean world, challenging the position of the cult of Asclepius as the chief center of religious healing. But Asclepius continued to retain his primacy. The popularity of the god owed much to his claim to be the god of both the rich *and* the poor. In a society conspicuously lacking in charitable concern for those in need, anyone who could not afford the fees of physicians could seek the aid of Asclepius. It was the god's claim that he cared for the poor, and he was satisfied with small thank offerings, which the poor could afford. In Roman times, the sanctuaries of Asclepius offered the hope of inexpensive healing for those who could not afford the services of a physician. Here the sick could spend long periods of convalescence. It is no wonder that Asclepius was called the most philanthropic of the gods and was regarded by early Christians as Christ's chief competitor. Some of his sanctuaries were still in existence in the sixth century AD.

There is little evidence of magical practices (incantations and the like) in secular medicine from Homer to Galen. Sophocles says that a good physician does not sing incantations over pains that should be cured by cutting. The writer of *The Sacred Disease* speaks disapprovingly of "magicians, purifiers, charlatans, and quacks," who resort to purifications and incantations in treating epilepsy. Yet the Greeks, like every other people in antiquity (and many today), believed in magic. Magical practices were almost certainly employed for healing, particularly when naturalistic methods were unsuccessful. Certain herbs were widely believed to possess magical healing properties. And impotence was believed to be the result of sorcery or malign magic. According to Diodorus, everyone resorts to incantations and prayers when the art of the physician fails to cure.[18] While not all physicians were free from magical practices and some employed incantations and recommended the use of amulets, these physicians were probably in a minority. In this regard Greek medicine differs from medicine in Egypt and Mesopotamia, where there was no definite boundary between magic and medicine.

Chapter Three

Rome

According to tradition, the city of Rome was founded in 753 BC. For the first 244 years (753–509 BC), in the conventional chronology, Rome was ruled by kings, and for the last century (616–509 BC) it was under the rule of its northern neighbors, the Etruscans. In 509 BC the Romans expelled the last of their Etruscan kings and gained their independence. They established a republic, governed by an oligarchy that exercised power through the Senate, which would last until 31 BC. Expansionist by nature, the Romans dominated Italy by 264 BC, then extended their power throughout the Mediterranean, which they conquered by 121 BC. Roman conquest of the Greek-speaking East brought a heterogeneous population of Greeks, Egyptians, and Near Eastern peoples under Roman rule. A series of civil wars from 88 to 31 BC led to dissolution of the republic and the establishment of the principate, a disguised absolute monarchy, by a grandnephew of Julius Caesar, Octavian, who became the first emperor of Rome under the adopted name Augustus. We refer to the period that Augustus inaugurated as the Roman Empire (31 BC–AD 476 or 493). The end of the civil wars brought about the two-hundred-year Pax Romana (Roman Peace), the longest continuous period of peace in the history of the Western world. Under expansionist emperors the Roman Empire spread from the Rhine-Danube frontier to the Sahara Desert and from Britain to the Euphrates River, bringing prosperity, ease of travel, the rule of law, and the fruits of Greco-Roman civilization to a population of more than 60 million. The empire was divided in two in AD 395, with the Western Empire falling to repeated attacks of nomadic tribes, chiefly Germanic, by AD 493. The Eastern Empire survived and was gradually transformed into the Byzantine Empire, which lasted until 1453, when it was conquered by the Ottoman Turks.

The Early Republic

Under the republic (509–31 BC) the practice of religion in Rome, as in Greece, was largely, but by no means exclusively, an official activity for the whole community. Its roots, which were agricultural and pastoral, furnished the economic and social background of the Romans. The Romans believed that they were surrounded by numina, supernatural beings initially conceived of as spiritual powers of a vague and undefined nature. Later these spirits were personified, and Roman religion, originally animistic, developed into polytheism. Even then they evoked no personal devotion, for they were gods of the state. The Romans believed themselves to be under the care of certain gods of the Greek and Roman pantheon (e.g., Jupiter, Juno), whose worship they maintained as a civic cult.

The official religion of Rome was supported by public funds and administered by magistrates and elected priests, who maintained traditional rituals and had charge of the temples. It was the duty of each citizen to take part in public worship, the purpose of which was to maintain the *pax deorum*, "the peace of the gods," which was the gods' continued favor and blessings on Rome. To this end, scrupulous observance of every traditional ritual was required. The civic cult was based on the idea of a contract between the community and the gods to the advantage of both. This contractual relationship was summarized by the Latin words *do ut des*, "I give in order that you may give [in return]." The Romans approached the gods with fear and reverence rather than with affection; they were so concerned with proper form that their worship tended to be mechanical and formal. In addition to the great divinities that protected Rome, the Romans worshiped the spirits and numina that protected their households or presided over some aspect of their lives. They assigned a spirit to every object or activity, and out of the many numina, each Roman would appease or seek the protection of those most relevant to his or her situation.

The Romans believed that if religious duties were neglected or carried out in a faulty manner, the gods might withdraw their favor or express their displeasure by sending disasters or prodigious events. Hence they took great care to provide regular festivals and to maintain the accustomed prayers and sacrifices to the gods. If a calamity or natural disaster occurred, it was generally regarded as a sign of divine retribution that required some sort of expiation in order to restore the *pax deorum*. The Romans lived in constant fear of displeasing some divinity. Divination was an important aspect of Roman religion, and for this purpose colleges of augurs and haruspices (Etruscan soothsayers) had the duty of discovering, by observing certain signs, whether the gods approved of a proposed action. In the case of an existing or pending disaster, such as famine, pestilence, or war, the Roman Senate might order additional sacrifices, supplications, vows, or other measures to avert the wrath of the gods. They were usually undertaken after consulting the augurs or haruspices or sacred books.

Although they tended to assign a separate deity to each function, the early Romans appear to have had no specific gods of either disease or healing. Rather, they relied on a variety of gods to protect them from disease. Thus Mars, the god of war, is appealed to in an early Latin hymn, the Carmen Arvale, not to permit any plague to come upon the Romans. And in an ancient prayer preserved by Cato the Elder (234–149 BC), Mars is called upon for protection from visible and invisible diseases and to bring health and strength to home and family.[1] Certain deities were frequently appealed to specifically in matters of health. The many household gods included a god for every function of the body and for every symptom of disease. For example, Carna, an Italian goddess of the underworld, had special care of the vital organs. She was asked to preserve the liver, the heart, and other organs, and she practiced magic that Romans could employ to avert disease.

Since it was not always possible for Romans to determine which numen or god had sent a plague, the generic formula "whether you be a god or goddess" was sometimes employed in prayers to avert the disease. The Romans also personified disease, hoping to appease it with worship and sacrifice and so avoid its further spread. Thus Febris (Fever) became a goddess who was thought to be favorable to humankind and to provide magical remedies for disease. Three temples were built in her honor in Rome. Other personifications of disease included Cloacina and Mefitis, who were invoked for protection and healing from vapors and poisonous gases.

For much of their early history, the Romans explained disease and disaster as the result of supernatural causation: the gods had been offended, and it was necessary that they be propitiated. As early as the reign of the Etruscan king Servius Tullius (traditionally dated 578–535 BC), prodigies (omens) occurred, accompanied by a pestilence, that the Romans regarded as the result of the neglect of certain religious rites. In 462 BC, when Rome was attacked by plague, the Senate ordered the people to beseech the gods to remit the disease. Widespread pestilence was responsible for the introduction of a number of foreign deities from Greece and elsewhere when Rome's own gods failed to avert disease. In 431 BC a temple was dedicated to Apollo in recognition of his aid in ending a plague that had raged for two years. Worshiped as Apollo Medicus (Apollo the Physician), over time he replaced many of the traditional Roman gods as averters of sickness and was even credited with discovering the art of healing. His cult later spread throughout the Latin West.

In 293 BC, when pestilence began to spread among the population of Rome, the Sibylline Books (the sacred oracles of the Romans) were consulted. They recommended that an embassy be sent to Epidaurus to bring the god Asclepius to Rome to end the disease. It was not until 291 BC, however, that the Romans sent the delegation. Although the priests at Epidaurus hesitated to honor the request, the god himself, in the form of a serpent, appeared in the temple before making his way to the ship that carried him to Rome. The serpent disembarked at Tiber Island, near the center of the city, and it was on that spot that the Romans dedicated a temple to him as Aesculapius in the same year. The cult of Aesculapius apparently was not prominent in Rome during the republican period, that is, until the end of the first century BC. But the introduction of his worship was nevertheless significant, for Aesculapius was viewed not merely as an averter of disease, like Apollo, but as a healer of individuals. In imperial times slaves were often abandoned on Tiber Island, where they could seek healing when they were too old or too sick to be profitable to their owners. If they recovered, they were given their freedom.

During the late republic, several other foreign gods of healing were introduced into Rome, offering healing by the use of magic, divination, or incubation, but we know little about them. The healing practices of Aesculapius in Rome were apparently quite similar to those of Greece. Sacred serpents and dogs were kept at his sanctuary, and although the practice of incubation is not mentioned before the end of the first century AD, it is likely that it was employed earlier. Inscriptions recording cases of healing have been found, but they date from the second century AD. They involve dream oracles, and the suggested remedies are of a theurgic (miracle-working) nature. The cult of Aesculapius came to enjoy great popularity in the first century AD and eventually spread throughout the West. Large numbers of votive offerings have been found at his sanctuary in Rome. The use of magic seems to have been a characteristic of healings by Aesculapius, probably representing an adaptation of the cult to Roman practices.

Until the migration of Greek physicians to Rome, the Romans, like the Hebrews, apparently had neither physicians nor secular medicine. Pliny the Elder says that for six hundred years they were "without physicians . . . but not without medicine." He explains this absence by stating that "it was not medicine itself that the forefathers condemned, but the medical profession, chiefly because they refused to pay fees to profiteers in order to save their lives."[2] Plague was averted by propitiating the gods. In individual cases of illness the Romans employed a combination of magical incantations and divination, much of which was inherited from the Etruscans and the Sabines, with folk remedies. The paterfamilias, who was the oldest living male in the family and the head of the household, usually acted as the de facto physician for members of the household. Typical of these practitioners of Roman popular medicine was Cato the Elder, who made himself familiar with medical matters so that he could treat his own family. Plutarch says that Cato

> had compiled a book of recipes and used them for the diet or treatment of any members of his household who fell ill. He never made his patients fast, but allowed them to eat herbs and morsels of duck, pigeon, or hare. He maintained that this diet was light and thoroughly suitable for sick people, apart from the fact that it often produced nightmares, and he claimed that by following it he kept both himself and his family in perfect health.[3]

Cato gives a good deal of medical advice in his handbook on agriculture, *De agricultura*. He includes many folk remedies that he probably derived, directly or indirectly, from the Italian peasantry. They are mingled with supplications, prayers, sacrifices, and ritual processions for the protection of his family, crops, and herds. He made much use of treatments containing cabbage, which he considered a panacea, and he regularly employed magical incantations.

For the early Romans every aspect of life—conception, gestation, birth, growth, marriage, and childbearing—was under the protection of a god or numen, whose protection they routinely sought. There were several native spirits or goddesses to whom a Roman matron could appeal for protection in childbirth, but most of these were eventually replaced by either Juno Lucina or Diana. Women recited magical formulas or incantations to ensure a safe childbirth and sometimes employed a ceremony of laying on hands, which was a means of transferring the power of a god or goddess for healing or, in the case of childbirth, for a safe delivery. The right hand was applied, signifying a good influence. A curious prophylactic ceremony, going back to primitive times, took place on the Roman festival of the Lupercalia, held in honor of the god Faunus. The priests of Faunus, clad only in goatskins, ran around the Palatine Hill, in the center of Rome, striking women with strips of goatskin to promote fertility.

The Late Republic

The first person said to have practiced medicine in Rome as a distinct profession was the Greek Archagathus, a wound specialist who settled in Rome in 219 BC and was given Roman citizenship. He was treated with great respect, but his excessive use of surgery and cautery eventually made him unpopular. He came to be called *carnifex*, "executioner," and he aroused disgust with the entire medical profession. He is unlikely to have been the first physician to practice at Rome but was probably the first civic physician who was paid a salary by the state. There was a demand for Greek physicians in Rome, and they continued to come.

Cato distrusted the Greeks, describing them in a letter to his son as "a quite worthless people, and an intractable one, and you must consider my words prophetic." He wrote: "When that race gives us its literature it will corrupt all things, and even all the more if it sends hither its physicians. They have conspired together to murder all foreigners with their physic, but this very thing they do for a fee, to gain credit and destroy. . . . I have forbidden you to have dealings with physicians."[4] Cato was unusual in his nativist opposition to Greek medicine, however, and Greek physicians enjoyed considerable popularity in Rome.

In the first century BC, the physician Asclepiades gained a wide reputation, which he passed on to his successors. The cult of Aesculapius also attracted adherents, and by the time of the empire it had appealed to the upper classes and even to emperors. But the traditional Roman practices of magic and folk medicine continued to exist even after the introduction of religious healing and secular medicine from Greece. This is illustrated by the compilation of folk and magical remedies made by the Roman naturalist Pliny the Elder (AD 23/4–79) in his encyclopedic *Natural History*. Romans also continued to consult soothsayers when ill.

The religious beliefs and general culture of the Romans underwent a significant change in the last two centuries before Christ, mainly as a result of Rome's conquest of Greece and the eastern Mediterranean. The upper classes tended to abandon traditional religion for either skepticism or philosophy, usually Stoicism or Epicureanism. Many ordinary people no longer found satisfaction in the worship of the traditional Roman gods. It was too formal and mechanical to satisfy the emotional needs of Romans who had left farming for the cities. As Rome conquered the Mediterranean world, soldiers returned from foreign campaigns and large numbers of captives poured into Italy as slaves. Many, especially those captured in the Eastern campaigns, brought with them foreign beliefs. Astrology, which had initially spread from Babylon to Greece, was influential in Italy by the first century AD. The belief was common that one's destiny was fixed at birth by the stars.

Magic too began to enjoy great vogue in Rome. Although the Roman author Pliny the Elder states that no one doubts that magic had its origin in medicine, there is no evidence that there was ever a connection between the two in Greece. Amulets had always been worn to ward off disease and personal disaster, but in general the practice of medicine in Greece and Rome was devoid of magical elements. The greatest Roman jurist, Ulpian (d. AD 228), in discussing the qualifications necessary to sue for unpaid remuneration for services, commented regarding physicians: "But one must not include people who make incantations or imprecations or, to use the common expression of imposters, exorcisms. For these are not branches of medicine, even though people exist who forcibly assert that such people have helped them."[5] Ulpian did not deny that alternative healing practices might prove efficacious in some circumstances, but he made it clear that those who called themselves physicians were not effective physicians or even physicians at all if their treatment involved magic or exorcism. As a result of Eastern influences, magicians became popular at Rome in the first century AD; they sold charms to curse enemies, exorcise demons, and heal diseases. The belief that certain animals, plants, and precious stones possessed occult properties that released magical forces through manipulation influenced healing practices.

Perhaps the most striking phenomenon of Roman religious life was the penetration of Italy and the western Mediterranean by a group of cults known as the mystery religions. They were religions that came from Egypt and Asia but had been modified by their contact with Greek civilization after Alexander's conquest of the Persian Empire. Once the mystery religions migrated to Rome, they quickly displaced Roman traditional religion, for they provided a personal satisfaction that the old formal religion was unable to offer. They featured elaborate rituals that appealed to the emotional needs of their adherents, and they offered the promise of immortality through personal communion with a god. They had a universal appeal to all classes, rich and poor, slave and free, citizen and foreigner. The most influential cults were those of the Great Mother (Magna Mater) and Cybele from Asia Minor, the Egyptian gods Isis and Serapis, and the Persian god Mithra. All offered cures, but the Egyptian gods specialized in healing. Isis was often associated with Asclepius, and incubation was practiced in her temples,

where painted tablets testified to miraculous cures. Those who sought her healing were required to confess their sins beforehand. But the mystery cults were
not alone in offering cures. Altogether more than one hundred healing shrines
could be found in Italy, many of them near mineral springs and associated with
deities and spirits of the natural world.

Medicine in the Roman Empire

The Roman Empire, which by the end of the first century BC spanned the
entire Mediterranean, became an amalgam of religious traditions whose variety
was reflected in their diverse approaches to healing. Healing played an important
part in many of the mystery cults, whose priests employed several means to cure
the sick, including astrology, magic, divination, and the use of herbs. Besides
Aesculapius, the most prominent of the Hellenistic healing gods was Serapis,
whose methods of healing were much like those of his rival Aesculapius. The
priests of the mystery cults came to exercise a strong influence over the adherents of their faith. They were versed in sacred knowledge and were looked to for
spiritual guidance by a society whose members increasingly were unable to live
without the aid of sacerdotal religion. The mystery religions placed great importance on mysterious methods of purification, whether through the performance
of rituals or through mortification and penance. In the late empire, magic played
a new role in therapeutics. Roman traditional medicine, of course, contained
some elements of magic that had established themselves through long use in
folk medicine. But the new influences were clearly of Eastern derivation and
appealed to the interest in occult approaches that characterized paganism in the
late Roman Empire.

Although physicians were widely available during the Roman imperial period, their social status varied enormously from that of highly educated physicians, whose patients were wealthy, to that of slaves. They were often, but not
always, associated with one or another medical sect and were dependent in a
society without medical licensure on a reputation based on their success in treating those who sought their help. They had been regarded as sufficiently valuable
to society to be granted financial benefits and civic honors by Greek cities in
the Hellenistic period to encourage them to establish or retain residence. In the
first century BC, Julius Caesar granted Roman citizenship to free physicians who
lived in Rome, and this act was followed by their being granted immunity from
taxes. It became increasingly difficult to distinguish between Greek and Roman

medicine. Perhaps one should speak instead of a continuum whose complexities indicate more than merely a Roman assimilation of Greek ideas.

Medicine in the Western Empire continued to be practiced largely by Greek physicians.[6] Most physicians who practiced in the West were either freedmen or slaves. It was not easy to determine the effects of any treatment, and physicians often disagreed with one another in what was a highly competitive marketplace. When confronted with chronic disorders that were painful but not fatal, physicians could do little. For this reason they usually declined to treat patients whose cases they considered hopeless, fearing damage to the reputation on which their practice rested. Many sick persons treated themselves for common ailments that they or a family member could alleviate by employing traditional remedies, or they relied on dreams for guidance. Yet despite all the resources available in the classical world, it is doubtful that physicians' ability to heal advanced appreciably from the fourth century BC to the second century AD.

Medicine and religious healing were complementary systems. The competition among healers of all kinds offered the sick person a multitude of opportunities for therapy. Geoffrey Lloyd identifies five "demarcated groups" of healers in the classical world: root cutters (Gk., *rhizitomoi*; L., *herbarii*), drug sellers (*pharmakopōlai*), midwives (Gk., *maiai*; L., *obstetrices*), religious healers, and learned physicians. Vivian Nutton's list is longer: herb cutters, druggists, midwives, gymnastic trainers (L., *iatraliptae*), diviners, exorcists, and priests.[7] Some—but not all—sick persons sought therapy from different healers because they attributed their illnesses to different etiologies.

For those who could afford them, physicians were ordinarily the healers from whom the sick sought treatment. While folk healers who offered amulets, herbs, and help from astrology were abundant, home remedies, administered within the family or by relatives and friends, may have been the most common form of medical therapy. But the healers who are visible in our sources were not folk healers but physicians. No professional organization or official body existed to separate the quack from the competent professional. To receive Roman citizenship under Julius Caesar or his successor, Augustus, the physician was required only to appear before a magistrate and affirm that he was a physician. No examination of training or professional qualifications was required. The competence and therapy offered varied from physician to physician. Some were highly trained and had adopted one or another theoretical approach, while others had little or no medical training and would be considered incompetent or charlatans both by their own professional colleagues and by a lay public that was often highly literate medically.

In assessing how many people had access to medical treatment by physicians, we must make geographical, class, and urban-rural distinctions. Physicians congregated in towns, to the disadvantage of rural dwellers. It was urbanization as much as the spread of Greek physicians throughout the Roman Empire that made medical care widely available. Cities like Rome and Constantinople had an abundance of medical specialists, yet even small towns might boast a surprisingly large number of physicians, as did Metapontum, in southern Italy, which had sixteen. The sick who lived on the edges of the empire were less well served. But even the most remote boundary areas attracted physicians, most of them probably serving with the Roman legions, who brought with them the medical traditions of the Greek world, as did a doctor by the name of Antiochus, who penned an elegant dedication to the healing gods Asclepius, Hygeia, and Pankeia in Chester, Britain, on the far-northern fringe of the empire.[8]

Under the Roman Empire, Greco-Roman medicine was, in theory and practice, Greek medicine that had been transported to Rome. With the Roman conquest of the Greek-speaking eastern Mediterranean in the last two centuries BC, thousands of Greeks were brought back to Rome as prisoners of war or as slaves.[9] That number included many Greek physicians, since the Roman upper classes had come to value Greek medicine. Medicine in the Western Empire was largely practiced by Greek physicians. While the social status of physicians was often high in the Greek East, it was much lower in the West. Their social background did not, however, prevent some physicians from penetrating the highest circles of Roman life—as court physicians, for example.

Of all the Greek physicians practicing medicine in Rome, the most distinguished was Galen. The last and greatest medical scientist of antiquity, he exercised an unparalleled influence on the development of medicine. Galen (129–c. 217) was born in Pergamum (modern Bergama, Turkey), an important city in western Asia Minor, the only son of Nikon, an architect and geometer. He was educated by his father until the age of fourteen, when he began to attend lectures in philosophy. When Galen was sixteen, his father decided that he should become a physician and thereafter spared no expense in his education. After studying under prominent medical teachers in Pergamum, Galen traveled to Smyrna in western Asia Minor, Corinth in Greece, and Alexandria in Egypt to study medicine.

At the age of twenty-eight he returned to Pergamum, where he was appointed physician to the school of gladiators. This position provided him with broad medical experience that laid the foundation for his later career. In 161 Galen left Pergamum for Rome, where he established a reputation as a successful physician and became acquainted with many prominent individuals. He returned to Pergamum in 166, claiming as the reason the envy of his colleagues, but it was more probably to escape a severe plague. Shortly after his return, however, he was summoned by the emperor Marcus Aurelius to Aquileia, at the head of the Adriatic, where he was engaged in preparations for war against the Germans. Galen followed the emperor to Rome in 169 and avoided further military service by gaining appointment as physician to the emperor's son Commodus. His position gave him the leisure to pursue medical research, writing, and lecturing, which he did with great success. Not much is known of Galen's later career. He continued to attend Commodus after he ascended the throne in 180, and he also attended Septimius Severus, who became emperor in 193. The date of Galen's death is uncertain. One source states that he died at the age of seventy, which would have been about 200. However, according to Arab biographers, he lived to be over eighty, which would make his death later than 210.

Galen was one of the most prolific authors of classical antiquity. He wrote more than 400 treatises, all of them in Greek. Many of his works have been lost, including a large number of his philosophical treatises that were destroyed in a fire in the Temple of Peace at Rome in 191. Nearly 140 works that have survived either in whole or in part are attributed to Galen. Some are of doubtful genuineness, and others are spurious. Still other works, while lost in Greek, are extant in Latin and Arabic translations. His writings are extremely diverse. They include works on anatomy, pathology, therapeutics, hygiene, dietetics, pharmacy, grammar, ethics, and logic, as well as commentaries on Hippocrates and Aristotle. Most of his extant works deal with medicine. Galen wrote clear Attic Greek, but he was prolix and diffuse, and his works are not easy to read. Moreover, he was vain, tactless, and quarrelsome, and his writings are often characterized by a polemical tone.

Galen's writings reveal a strong teleological emphasis. He believed that everything had been made by the Creator (or Demiurge) for a divine purpose and that the entire creation bears witness to his benevolence. In his treatise *On the Usefulness of the Parts of the Human Body* Galen expresses the belief that true piety lies in recognizing and explaining the wisdom, power, and excellence of the Creator rather than in offering a multitude of sacrifices. He accepted the Aristotelian principle that nature does nothing in vain, and he attempted to show that every human organ was designed to serve a particular function. He believed that in the minutest detail the human body exhibits its divine design.

Although Galen believed in one god, his depiction of him as a divine crafts-man was drawn not from Judeo-Christian sources but from Plato's *Timaeus*, as was his argument from design. He criticized Moses for holding (in the Creation narrative in Genesis) the doctrine of *creatio ex nihilo* (creation from nothing) and the belief that nature originated as an act of God's sovereign will. Galen was acquainted with both Jews and Christians, and he refers to their beliefs several times in his philosophical and medical works. He was the first pagan writer to treat Christianity with respect as a philosophy rather than, as most educated Romans did, as a superstitious sect. He admired Christians for their contempt of death, their sexual purity, their self-control in regard to food and drink, and their pursuit of justice, in all of which he regarded them as not inferior to pagan philosophers. He criticized Christians and Jews, however, for their refusal to base their doctrines on reason rather than solely on faith and revealed authority. In the late second century AD a group of Roman Christians in Asia Minor led by Theodotus of Byzantium attempted to formulate Christianity in philosophical terms. They are said to have admired Galen, and it is likely that they were influenced by his philosophical works. They taught an adoptionist Christology (the view that Christ was merely the adopted son of God), and for this and other heresies they were excommunicated by church authorities.

Galen enjoyed an enviable reputation in his own time both as a physician and as a philosopher. Soon after his death he came to be recognized as the greatest of all medical authorities. His eclecticism, which permitted him to take what was best from all medical sects, his claim to reproduce the ideas of Hippocrates, the encyclopedic comprehensiveness of his medical works, and his greatness as a scientist were largely responsible for his influence. Because his writings were voluminous, they were summarized in handbooks, synopses, and medical encyclopedias. The pre-Galenic medical sects gradually disappeared and were replaced by an all-embracing Galenic system that united medicine and philosophy and would dominate medicine for more than a millennium. As anatomical and physiological research ceased in late antiquity, medicine became increasingly scholastic and was taught from a selection of Galen's works.

Galen's direct influence was initially greater in the Byzantine East, where his ideas were preserved in medical encyclopedias, than in the Latin West. In the ninth century many of his works were collected and translated into Arabic and

Syriac by Hunayn ibn Ishāq (808–873), a Nestorian Christian Arab physician, and his school. In the course of the eleventh century they were translated from Arabic into Latin and Hebrew, and they came to dominate medicine in the West just as they had dominated Byzantine and Arabic medicine. Galen's authority was regarded as second only to Aristotle's. Although a pagan, Galen appealed equally to Jews, Muslims, and Christians, who found his teleology and monotheism compatible with their own faiths. The appearance of his collected Greek works in the sixteenth century spurred new interest in Galen and led to a revival of medical experimentation. It was during the Renaissance that his reputation reached its apex, but it soon began to be challenged by new discoveries, particularly in the fields of anatomy and physiology. Nevertheless, ideas championed by Galen, particularly his formulation of humoral pathology, continued to influence medical practice until the nineteenth century.

Healing Cults

Most religions included an element of religious healing, which was intended to complement rather than to compete with secular medicine. Healing shrines, like miracle workers, were probably not the first choice of most who needed medical help (except the very poor), but they were often the last resort for those who found no help from physicians. In the Roman Empire those who desired supernatural healing could seek help from a variety of gods, goddesses, demigods, and heroes. Undoubtedly the most important was Asclepius (the Roman Aesculapius). By the second century of the Christian era he was the healing god par excellence, worshiped either alone or in conjunction with other gods at 732 temples and shrines, 670 of them in the Mediterranean world.[10] These shrines were not merely centers of worship; they were sites to which pilgrims traveled for healing, much as they visit Lourdes, Fatima, or Guadalupe today.

As the most common form of divine healing in the classical world, incubation was a feature of a number of cults besides that of Asclepius, including the mystery religions. By the end of the second century AD incubation was employed by many gods, both Greek (e.g., Hygieia and Pan) and Eastern (e.g., Isis and Serapis).[11] To potential converts, one of the greatest attractions of these deities was their claim to be able to heal. Their temples complemented existing shrines of local heroes and sacred springs that had drawn the sick to nearby sites for centuries. Healing cults advertised their cures by aretalogies (public testimonies) of pilgrims who had been healed, such as the *iamata* displayed at the shrines of Asclepius. These aretalogies, though often formulaic, were sufficiently convincing to draw those who could not obtain healing through secular medicine. It has been suggested that healing shrines, particularly those of Asclepius, were popular in Roman times, in part because they promised healing without charge to the poor, who could not afford the services of a physician. But they did not serve the poor alone. Those who suffered from chronic or incurable conditions were frequent pilgrims at healing sites.

One of the most interesting ancient accounts of healing by Asclepius comes from the writings of the celebrated Greek rhetorician and neurotic hypochondriac Aelius Aristides (AD 117–89 or 129–89), who spent much of his life in the pursuit of personal health. Aristides was the son of a wealthy country gentleman in Asia Minor. He was educated in Pergamum and Athens and studied under the same teacher who taught the future emperor Marcus Aurelius. He became a celebrated sophist and lecturer and traveled the length and breadth of the Roman Empire. He was much in demand to give ceremonial speeches as well as eulogies in leading cities, including Rome, Athens, and Smyrna, and to deliver formal compliments to the emperor. At the age of twenty-six, with a brilliant career ahead of him, he suffered the first of a series of illnesses that made him an invalid for some twelve years. He tells us that after a difficult journey to Rome in the winter of 143/144, during which he suffered from asthma, fever, earache, and toothache, he spent much of his time in a dark room wrapped in woolen blankets. He described his illnesses in a journal, the *Sacred Tales*, which fills five volumes of more than three hundred thousand lines and is the most fascinating autobiographical document we have from the ancient world of a deeply religious but chronically ill man and his attempts to find healing. He returned to Asia Minor, and in 146 he visited the sanctuary of Asclepius, where he believed that the god spoke to him. Aristides became a devoted servant of Asclepius, whose help he believed he had often received. In his journal Aristides recorded conversations with the god as well as visions, predictions, and oracles.

By the second century AD, Pergamum, in Asia Minor, had replaced Epidaurus as the chief center of healing by Asclepius. Miraculous healing by the god gave way to therapeutics that were in many respects not very different from those that a contemporary physician might prescribe. Pilgrims received in a dream detailed instructions from the god for pursuing a particular regimen or a medical remedy for their illness. Asclepius's priests often recommended to incubants practical regimens of gymnastics, swimming, riding, fasting, diet, and purgatives, as well as more exceptional treatments. But, as revealed in Aristides's *Sacred Tales*, the regimens they recommended sometimes included fantastic prescriptions, such as swimming in a cold stream in winter. Aristides's illnesses were of a familiar psychosomatic type that included asthma, headaches, insomnia, and digestive troubles. He records that in his dreams he met Asclepius on several occasions. The prescriptions the god gave him were both penitential in nature and self-inflicted torments, though they have parallels among ascetic groups in antiquity, for example: "He is made to forswear hot baths for more than five years, compelled to run barefoot in winter, to take river baths in the frost and mudbaths in an icy wind, and even to make himself seasick."[12]

During his lifetime he remained the devoted servant of the god, who became not merely a divine healer but an intimate adviser in every aspect of his life, as well as a divine companion with whom Aristides came to feel a sense of spiritual unity. While his experience remains unique in our accounts of the devotees of Asclepius, we are told that the god appeared to many people both in healing and in forecasting their future. And no less distinguished personages than the emperor Marcus Aurelius, who writes that the gods gave him dreams that cured his illnesses, and Galen, who relates that Asclepius helped him as a physician to save lives through divine dreams, testify to the fact that some of the best-educated men of the day believed in the healing dreams of Asclepius.

Demons and Demonism in Late Antiquity

In Mesopotamia and Egypt belief in demons was an important part of the religious framework, and diseases were often attributed to them. This was not true in Greece and Rome, however. It has been argued that a belief in the power and influence of demons entered the classical world in the second century AD and that it became widespread in late antiquity. This phenomenon, the so-called daimonization of religion, has been largely taken for granted in discussions of late Roman religion, both pagan and Christian. According to the conventional theory, in the third century AD "philosophy and folk-belief, instead of progressing along separate pathways, 'joined hands' in a common belief in demons which Christianity then transformed altogether into evil spirits." This theory remains the dominant narrative, and it informs many modern historical accounts of the intellectual atmosphere of the late Roman Empire. Thus Peter Brown writes that a perceived ubiquity of demons was one of the elements of the "new mood" that spread rapidly in the age of the Antonine emperors (AD 138–80) and brought about a spiritual revolution that came to characterize late antiquity. Several scholars, however, have challenged the theory as lacking in evidence. And when closely examined, it does not seem very convincing. Arthur Darby Nock argued that Greco-Roman society in late antiquity was not demon-ridden, or at least not more so than any other period of antiquity. Possession and exorcism were not new, while remedies such as amulets and purifications had long been readily available to guard against demons. In any event, the perceived existence of hostile demons was no worse than that of the traditional gods, who had always needed to be appeased.[13]

The question when, if at all, the alleged daimonization of religion in the Roman Empire occurred has several possible answers, among them the following: (1) The second and third centuries witnessed an increasing belief in the activity of demons; this increase was either (*a*) rapid or (*b*) gradual, reaching its peak in the fourth and fifth centuries. (2) The second and third centuries saw no increase in belief in the activity of demons, since belief in demons had long existed in the Greco-Roman world. Of these possibilities, the theory that there was a gradual increase in the belief in demons in late antiquity (1*b*) seems to best fit the evidence we have. The commonly held view of a rapid increase in the belief in demons in the second and third centuries (1*a*) relies less on contemporary evidence than on an assumed trajectory that traces the prominence of belief in demons in the fourth and fifth centuries back to discussions among both pagans and Christians of the second century. Scholars such as Peter Brown exaggerate both the ubiquity and the influence of demonic belief in late antiquity.[14] There is little, if any, evidence from contemporary sources to support the theory that pagans or Christians attributed disease to demons. In fact, that view assumes both that Christians adopted a Jewish demonic theory of disease etiology and that demonology grew rapidly in the second and third centuries. Neither is supported by the evidence. Third-century medical theories of the etiology of disease were not demonic etiologies, and we have no reason to think that educated popular opinion differed from medical opinion in that regard.

Ludwig Edelstein has demonstrated that demons had virtually no connection with Greco-Roman medicine. It would be difficult, he observes, to find a physician who accepted a theory of demonic etiology. Physicians unanimously rejected it and treated the explanation with disdain. Nor does Edelstein find any philosophers who accepted demonic etiology of disease, not even among the Neoplatonists of late antiquity, who adopted thaumaturgy (performing miracles). The Neoplatonist Plotinus (AD 205–269/70) heaps scorn on those who attribute disease to demons, arguing that disease is caused by natural factors and is healed by medical treatment. One might expect, however, that physicians and philosophers, who were educated, took for granted natural causation but that popular opinion would incline toward demonic explanations. But Edelstein argues that patients who believed that demons caused disease would not have sought the services of physicians because physicians attributed disease to natural causes. A doctor could not heal a disease that his patient thought demonically induced; the patient would have to consult a healer who claimed to be able to expel demons by magic or drugs that he and his patients believed would be efficacious against them. If the sick consulted physicians, it was because they expected them to be able to heal diseases that they had diagnosed by using natural explanations that their patients accepted, just as they accepted their prescribed therapies.

In two prominent religious traditions, however, we do find disease attributed to demons. The first is Gnosticism. According to Plotinus, the Gnostics asserted that diseases were spirit beings that could be expelled by magical formulas.[15] The other tradition is Judaism. In the postexilic period, after the resettlement of Palestine by Jews who returned from exile in Babylon in 538 BC, one begins to find reference to the activity of demons and exorcism in Jewish literature. Jewish exorcists used magical means, such as amulets, both to prevent and to cure disease, and they used exorcism, either by outward means or by formulas of incantation, to expel disease-causing demons. Both reflect syncretistic elements in Second Temple Judaism.

We know of several Jewish exorcists and magicians, the most prominent in Roman times being the Jewish exorcist Eleazar. Josephus records that he once saw him perform an exorcism in the presence of the emperor Vespasian (r. AD 69–79), his officers, and his troops. Eleazar placed a ring that held a root allegedly prescribed by Solomon near the nostrils of a demoniac. The demon was drawn out and commanded not to return as Eleazar recited the name of Solomon and uttered incantations attributed to him. In the Second Temple period Solomon came to be regarded as a celebrated magician and exorcist, based on his ostensible knowledge of the virtues of plants and animals and his power over spirits. He was said to have written incantations both to cure illnesses and to exorcise demons.[16]

The Jewish Essenes are also known to have practiced exorcism. They were famed for their skill in employing magic, exorcism, and folk medicine for healing. Several documents from the Qumran community, on the shores of the Dead Sea, attribute legendary afflictions of pagan kings to demons who were expelled by Jewish exorcists. In fact, Jewish exorcists enjoyed a favorable reputation among pagans throughout the Roman Empire. Jewish magical papyri dating from the second to the fifth centuries preserve a number of incantations and formulas of exorcism. Exorcists are mentioned on several occasions in the Gospels. It is difficult to estimate how widely first-century Jews outside sectarian groups like the Essenes and those who sought out Jewish exorcists believed in the demonic etiology of disease. Although that belief has left its mark on rabbinic literature, it was not the predominant view of disease among Palestinian Jews. And given its often sensational nature, it is likely to play a more prominent role in the surviving evidence than it played in fact.

There is no question that a heightened supernaturalism characterized late Roman society in the fourth and fifth centuries. But a past generation of scholars has overemphasized the influence of demons, magic, and miracles on the thought and practice of Roman pagans and Christians of late antiquity. While some literature of this period is indeed marked by a supernaturalistic tendency, most of it is not. Rational approaches to both medicine and religion continued to influence the thinking of a large proportion of ordinary people. Natural methods of healing continued to predominate in medicine. While folk medicine and religious healing, influenced by magic and astrology, were widely practiced, they complemented but did not replace secular medicine. There was, however, a broad array of sources of healing available to those who sought them.

Chapter Four

Early Christianity

Christianity originated within the framework of Palestinian Judaism. Its founder was Jesus of Nazareth (c. 4 BC–c. AD 30), who, in a public ministry that lasted about three years, announced the coming of God's kingdom, which had long been anticipated by the Jews. His ministry of preaching, teaching, and healing attracted wide popular attention, but it also drew opposition from religious leaders, which ended with his death by crucifixion. Three days after his death, a group of his followers in Jerusalem, led by the disciples he had gathered around him, proclaimed that he had risen from the dead. They viewed this as authentication of his claim to be the Jewish Messiah and the Son of God, and they believed that by his death he had atoned for the sins of his people.

Jesus's followers carried the new faith throughout Palestine, where they initially sought converts among fellow Jews. The earliest significant attempt to win gentile (non-Jewish) converts was made by the apostle Paul (d. c. AD 67). Following his conversion, Paul made several missionary journeys throughout the eastern Roman Empire and established churches in a number of important cities. By about AD 60 the new faith had been carried by Paul and Jesus's disciples to most regions of the eastern Mediterranean and as far west as Rome. By the middle of the second century there were small but thriving Christian communities in all major and many minor cities of the Roman Empire.

At first Christianity was regarded by the Roman government as a Jewish sect, and it benefited from special legal privileges enjoyed by the Jews. In AD 64, however, the emperor Nero, seeking a scapegoat to divert suspicion that he had set fire to Rome, accused the Christians of having done so and began actively to persecute them. For the next 250 years, Christians faced persecution, sometimes throughout the empire, sometimes locally and sporadically. The Romans regarded Christians as traitors for their refusal to offer sacrifice to the Roman emperor as a god, and as atheists for their failure to participate in public pagan worship. Rumor and demonization led to charges against them of cannibalism, incest, and hatred of humankind. Full-scale systematic persecution throughout the Roman Empire commenced in the third century, culminating in violent persecution under the emperor Diocletian that began in 303. In 313 the emperor Constantine, who in the previous year had converted to Christianity, issued, together with his coemperor, Licinius, the Edict of Milan, which ended persecution and made Christianity a legal religion for the first time.

The reign of Constantine (312–37) marked a significant turning point in the history of Christianity. With the exception of Julian the Apostate (r. 361–63), all subsequent Roman emperors professed Christianity and favored it in both policy and legislation. An alliance between church and state began that remained an enduring although sometimes tense and conflictive feature of Western Christianity throughout the Middle Ages. Constantine provided public support for the church, granted various immunities and privileges to the clergy, strengthened church law by imposing the force of civil sanctions, attempted to suppress heresy, and sought, by summoning a church council at Nicaea in 325, to settle a theological dispute between orthodox and Arian Christians over the question whether Jesus was God or a created being. Although paganism remained the official Roman religion for most of the fourth century, it gradually declined, until in 391 the emperor Theodosius closed pagan temples, forbade public pagan worship, and made Christianity the official Roman religion.

Another significant event of Constantine's reign was his removal of the capital of the empire to the Greek city Byzantium—which he renamed Constantinople—at the entrance to the Black Sea, in 330. In 395 the empire was permanently divided between East and West, and this political separation ultimately led to the division of the church. In spite of heresies and schisms, the church had hitherto remained institutionally unified, although the Western and Eastern branches had already begun in late antiquity to assume their own distinctive theological and cultural identities. After 395 they increasingly diverged, although the division between Eastern and Western Christianity was not made official until the

Great Schism of 1054, which formalized the break between what ultimately became the Orthodox churches in the East and the Catholic Church in the West.

Healing in the New Testament and the Early Church

On opening the pages of the New Testament, many modern readers find themselves in what appears to be an alien world, in which supernatural forces intervene in ordinary life. The Gospels focus on the extraordinary Palestinian ministry of Jesus, who casts out demons and miraculously heals the sick of every description. The book of Acts recounts the activities of Jesus's disciples, who themselves exercise miraculous healing and exorcism and carry their supernatural gifts throughout the Mediterranean world, a world in which they themselves encounter exorcists and magicians. If we were to describe early Christian beliefs regarding sickness and healing on the basis of a cursory reading of the Gospels and Acts, we might be inclined to summarize them as follows: Disease is caused by sin or by demons and can be healed supernaturally. Some illnesses can be cured only by exorcism, others by miraculous healing, and still others are susceptible to healing by prayer, faith, or anointing. With slight modification this description can be found in several standard studies of the role of medicine in the early Christian church, including those written by biblical, classical, and medical scholars. In fact, studied carefully and placed in the context of early Christian culture, the evidence points in a very different direction.

During his ministry of three years, for which the four Gospels constitute our major—and nearly only reliable—source, Jesus is said to have performed more than two dozen miracles of healing. The Gospels depict Jesus's miracles as "signs" (*ta semeia*) demonstrating his Messianic identity and indicating that the kingdom of God had come in fulfillment of Hebrew prophecy. In the Fourth Gospel, Jesus himself is said to have proclaimed his miracles to be an indication of his Messiahship. They are differentiated in the Gospels from the miracles performed by contemporary exorcists and magicians. While Jesus is said to have cast out demons, the Gospels distinguish between his acts of exorcism and his acts of healing.[1] It does not appear that either he or his disciples considered demons to be the cause of disease. Most of the symptoms described in the healing narratives of Jesus are those of ordinary diseases or congenital conditions for which a natural causation was assumed by those who had contracted them. Moreover, the Gospels distinguish the symptoms of ordinary disease from those that accompanied demonic possession, which usually manifested erratic or abnormal behavior.

A theme that appears often in the Gospels is Jesus's insistence that the love of God required the manifestation of personal charity toward one's fellows. It was a consistent feature of his attacks on the kind of religious formalism that emphasized religious ritual but ignored "the weightier matters of the law," namely, a love of one's fellows. In several passages in the Gospels, Jesus enunciates the pattern of personal charity that was to characterize his followers. "For I was hungry and you gave me food, I was thirsty and you gave me something to drink, I was a stranger and you welcomed me, I was naked and you gave me clothing, I was sick, and you took care of me [*epeskepsasthe*], I was in prison and you visited me. . . . Just as you did not do it to one of the least of these, you did not do it to me."[2]

In Jesus's teaching, love was to be extended not only to fellow believers but also to neighbors and even enemies. When Jesus was asked, "And who is my neighbor?" he responded by relating the parable of the Good Samaritan:

> Just then a lawyer [an expert in the Torah] stood up to test Jesus. "Teacher," he said, "what must I do to inherit eternal life?" He said to him, "What is written in the law? What do you read there?" He answered, "You shall love the Lord your God with all your heart, and with all your soul, and with all your strength, and with all your mind; and your neighbor as yourself." And he said to him, "You have given the right answer; do this, and you will live."
>
> But wanting to justify himself, he asked Jesus, "And who is my neighbor?" Jesus replied, "A man was going down from Jerusalem to Jericho, and fell into the hands of robbers, who stripped him, beat him, and went away, leaving him half dead. Now by chance a priest was going down that road; and when he saw him, he passed by on the other side. So likewise a Levite, when he came to the place and saw him, passed by on the other side. But a Samaritan while traveling came near him; and when he saw him, he was moved with pity. He went to him and bandaged his wounds, having poured oil and wine on them. Then he put him on his own animal, brought him to an inn, and took care of him. The next day he took out two denarii, gave them to the innkeeper, and said, 'Take care of him; and when I come back, I will repay you whatever more you spend.' Which of these three, do you think, was a neighbor to the man who fell into the hands of the robbers?" He said, "The one who showed him mercy." Jesus said to him, "Go and do likewise."[3]

In the parable, the Levite and the priest who passed the wounded man by and refused to give him assistance disgraced their own moral standards, which required them to care for their own. But Jesus went beyond Jewish concepts of charity, which were directed inward to one's own faith community. The novelty of Jesus's teaching was that beneficence extends beyond one's own community and indeed even to one's enemies. Jesus's command was to demonstrate compassion to the sick ("Go and do likewise"), not to offer miraculous healing. The parable of the Good Samaritan became the most iconic summons to the compassionate treatment of the sick in Christian medical philanthropy.[4]

That early Christians did not believe that miraculous healing was normative in the treatment of illness is suggested by the fact that outside the narratives of Jesus's healings one finds little reference to it in the New Testament. The book of Acts describes relatively few healings, which the writer attributes to Jesus's disciples (e.g., 8:3–10). They belong to the category of "signs and wonders" that confirm the disciples' apostolic credentials as authoritative interpreters of Jesus's message (see 14:3). The writer of Acts assumes that the diseases they healed were caused by natural conditions, and neither he nor those healed attribute them to demons. When we turn to the New Testament Epistles (most of which were written before the Gospels), we do not find any case of sickness that is either attributed to demonic causation or healed miraculously. While the miracles described in the Gospels were meant to demonstrate the advent of the Messianic age, first-century Christians appear not to have expected that it would result in the supernatural healing of their diseases.

There is only one discussion of religious healing in the Epistles. It is found in the epistle of James, perhaps the earliest of all New Testament writings, which was probably composed before AD 50. The epistle prescribes a rite of healing in which the presbyters (elders) of the local congregation anoint the sick and pray for their recovery, which is promised. The passage has been interpreted in a variety of ways. Does it refer to the restoration of physical health and recovery or to the healing of a spiritual condition? Although the weight of scholarly opinion favors the former, one might offer compelling arguments in support of the view that spiritual healing and restoration are the object. A few verses earlier James cites Job, who patiently endured his physical affliction, as an example for Christians to emulate.[5]

There are, moreover, indications in Acts and the Epistles that Christians in the apostolic age were rarely healed miraculously, while some, such as Paul's friend Epaphroditus (Phil. 2:25–27) and Trophimus (2 Tim. 4:20), were not healed at all. We cannot say whether either of these men was healed by religious means or even whether Trophimus recovered. Paul continued to suffer from his "thorn in the flesh" (2 Cor. 12:7–10), which may have been a physical disability that was never healed. The evidence, scattered and circumstantial as it is, suggests that first-century Christians relied on ordinary means of healing, such as conventional medicine or folk or traditional remedies. Paul's advice to Timothy to take a little wine for his stomach (1 Tim. 5:23) is an example of the latter.

It does not appear, in fact, that religious or faith healing replaced conventional medicine or even played a major role in the first four centuries of the Christian church. Leading Christian writers of the period exhibit almost universally positive views of medicine. Thus Origen (c. 185–c. 254) considered medicine "beneficial and essential to mankind,"[6] while Tertullian (c. 160–c. 225), who frequently employs medical analogies in his writings, believed that medicine was appropriate for Christians to use. The theme of Jesus the Great Physician (Christus medicus) was popular in the second century, though it was largely used in a metaphorical sense to describe Jesus as the Savior of sin-sick souls, not of physical healing. Indeed, medical care, far from being distrusted by early Christians, became for them a widely used model for the cure of the soul.

The early Christian understanding of disease combined both theological and medical elements. Christians regarded disease as merely one aspect of the material (rather than the moral) evil that had arisen from the Fall. Within the context of disease and healing that they had inherited from Judaism, Christians looked on illness as the result of natural, if providential, causes that could be treated by physicians or other healers, of whom a broad spectrum existed in the "medical marketplace" of the classical world. Christians broke bones and contracted the same diseases that their pagan and Jewish neighbors did, for which they ordinarily consulted physicians if they were available and if they could afford their services. When medical or natural means of healing were not available, they might seek healing by prayer. But in cases for which no relief was possible, Christians were advised to submit patiently to God's will. Early Christian writers repeatedly speak of suffering as one of God's means of producing spiritual maturity. Faith and trust in God could transform suffering into a positive experience and produce Christian graces such as humility, patience, and dependence on Christ.[7]

The widely held theodicy of the ancient world—that sin or failure to perform required religious rituals properly brought retribution often in the form of illness—was challenged by the early Christians, who formulated a view of the human condition in which suffering assumed a positive role that it had previously lacked. Christians believed that rather than bringing shame and disapproval, disease and sickness brought the sufferer a favored status that invited sympathy and compassionate care. In the classical world, neither philosophy nor religion encouraged a compassionate response to human suffering. During times of plague the sick and dying were abandoned, and corpses were often left unburied in order to prevent the spread of contagion, a scene most famously found in Thucydides's description of the Plague of Athens in the fifth century BC but echoed in other descriptions of plagues in antiquity. One example is the contemporary account by Dionysius, patriarch of Alexandria, of the Plague of Cyprian in the mid-third century AD:

> The heathen behaved in the very opposite way. At the first onset of the disease, they pushed the sufferers away and fled from their dearest, throwing them into the roads before they were dead, and treating unburied corpses as dirt, hoping thereby to avert the spread and contagion of the fatal disease; but do what they might, they found it difficult to escape.[8]

Christians viewed suffering as an opportunity to provide care of the sick and dying. At the same time, they saw in suffering an opportunity for personal self-examination that could bring spiritual illumination. While Christians believed that suffering might be God's chastisement for sin, they did not posit a simple direct correlation between sin and suffering. Rather, they viewed it as a means of grace for the spiritual benefit of the sufferer.

The Cause of Disease

Some scholars have maintained that early Christians rejected a naturalistic etiology of disease and that they regarded demons as the cause of all, or at any rate much, illness. While this interpretation is by no means accepted by all or even most New Testament scholars or historians of early Christianity, it can be said to be a currently dominant narrative. It is true that in the Second Temple period one sees frequent reference to the activity of demons and exorcism in Jewish literature. In the Gospels and in Acts, for example, one finds mention of them, among whom are the seven sons of Skevas, a Jewish chief priest.[9] Underlying the view that early Christians ascribed disease wholly or partly to demons is the assumption that the Gospel accounts of Jesus's exorcisms reflect contemporary Jewish views of demonology. The biblical evidence, however, does not suggest that Jesus shared the demonology of some of his Palestinian contemporaries, or even that most Palestinians attributed disease to demons.

Apart from three apparent cases in the Gospels,[10] the New Testament does not ascribe any illness or physical dysfunction to demons. A number of medical conditions that Jesus healed are described in the Gospels. They include deafness, muteness, blindness, leprosy, fever, dysentery, a uterine hemorrhage, lameness, paralysis, dropsy, and a withered hand. While no immediate cause is given for any of these illnesses or symptoms, most of those mentioned in the Gospels (indeed, in the New Testament) fall in the category of ordinary diseases or congenital conditions, none of them remarkable.

Moreover, the symptoms given for diseases or physical impairments are for the most part distinguished from the symptoms that are said typically to accompany demonic possession, such as erratic or self-destructive behavior. In most reported instances of illness, Jesus is said physically to have healed the sick person rather than to have expelled demons. It is, in fact, an important distinction of Jesus's treatment of the sick that he healed them rather than cast out demons. Jesus often healed chronic illness or longstanding conditions for which medical treatment had been unsuccessful.[11]

When we turn from the Gospels and Acts to the New Testament Epistles and the Apocalypse, we find that demonic possession is notable for its absence. In fact, apart from in the Gospels, demons are seldom alluded to in first- or early second-century Christian literature. That exorcism is not mentioned perhaps reflects the absence of perceived demonic possession in New Testament churches. Christian writers of the first two centuries associated the narratives of demonic activity in Jesus's time with his battle against the powers of Satan. They believed that after Jesus's resurrection demons continued to be present largely in the spiritual realm, especially as the active spiritual presences behind pagan idols. Tertullian asserted that any Christian could perform exorcisms.

In the late second century a rite of exorcism came to be administered to catechumens (new converts) before baptism to formally and liturgically separate them from the moral influence of evil that had dominated their lives before conversion. The churches did not believe that converts had been possessed, but that they had been under the spiritual influence of demons. And while we find several incidental references to sickness in the New Testament Epistles, they do not record a single instance of sickness that is either attributed to demons or healed miraculously. It is not until the mid- and late second century that we find demons mentioned in the legendary narratives of the Gnostic and Ecratite apocryphal gospels.

Early Christians, like the majority of their contemporaries, implicitly accepted a natural causality of disease within the framework of a Christian world-view. If they sometimes spoke in a manner that blurred the distinction between ultimate and proximate causation, it was because they believed that the presence of God was operative in natural forces. They viewed Jesus's exorcisms and miraculous healings as signs that the kingdom of God had entered history, not as normative models for the healing of ordinary disease. They sought out physicians to cure ordinary diseases and valued the healing power of medicine. In their view, however, medical treatment and prayer were not mutually exclusive but necessarily complementary. Some early Christians resorted to the use of amulets or relied on dreams, predictions, and portents, not because their faith encouraged them to do so (in fact, it explicitly forbade some of these means), but because they were commonly used in the broader culture of the Roman Empire. And where treatment had proven ineffective or few doctors were to be found, some likely had recourse to parallel therapies, consulting healers who employed magical or folk cures.

Christian Healing in Late Antiquity

In the latter half of the fourth century AD there was a pronounced increase in the number of Christian miracles reported in our sources, which are portrayed with marked sensationalism. The major source of this phenomenon was the Desert Fathers of the Eastern Roman Empire, beginning with Anthony (251?–356) and his disciple Pachomius (c. 290–346), who exercised widespread influence and whom popular legend credited with having performed many miracles. The Desert Fathers were generally orthodox (by the contemporary church's definition of orthodoxy). As their reputation for holiness and asceticism grew, some of them were sought out by ordinary Christians for spiritual counsel and physical healing. Their ability to heal was attributed to their holiness and to the control ascetics had over their own bodies through discipline and mortification.

Athanasius (c. 296–393) wrote in Greek a life of Anthony, the founder of anchoritic, or hermitic, monasticism, shortly after the latter's death in 356. It was soon translated into Latin, creating a new genre of literature known as hagiography. Lives of saints, such as Gregory of Nyssa's lives of Gregory Thaumaturgus and Saint Macrina, proliferated, inspired by the enormous popularity of Athanasius's work; they would constitute the most popular form of Christian literature in the late fourth and fifth centuries. These biographies described the miraculous exploits that were popularly attributed to the ascetics: casting out of demons, miraculous healing of diseases, and raising of the dead. The ascetics were said to effect miraculous cures by prayer, making the sign of the cross, laying their hands on the afflicted, or applying bread, oil, water, or garments that they had blessed.

Miracles of healing were also attributed to bishops like Ambrose (c. 337–397), the influential bishop of Milan.

With the veneration of ascetics, who could be looked to for healing, a new interest arose in martyrs and relics (the material remains of saints or objects related to them). The remains of the earliest Christian martyrs had been venerated because martyrs were thought to have been especially blessed by God, since they had proven their faith by their willingness to die for it. Hence their tombs were honored and attracted pilgrims, who began to attribute miracles and cures to these martyrs. The relics of saints or martyrs extended to posterity the benefits the saints had conferred on those in need during their own lifetime.

The influence of the new views is evident in the growing interest that miraculous healing came to have for Augustine (354–430), bishop of Hippo, in North Africa, the most important theologian in the Western church. Early in his Christian life Augustine accepted the common opinion that miracles no longer occurred, having ended with the age of the apostles. This view is explicitly stated in his treatise *Of True Religion*, penned in 390, in which he writes that men no longer need miraculous proofs of their faith that rely on the authority of scripture, since reason can now lead to understanding and knowledge of the truth and virtue. Augustine, in fact, ridiculed claims of contemporary miracles made by the unorthodox Donatist Christians of North Africa. Later in life he began to change his mind, particularly after the bones of the martyr Stephen were brought to Hippo in 424 and allegedly wrought some seventy miracles in less than two years. He collected accounts of these and other healings and cataloged a large number of them in book 22, chapter 8, of *The City of God*. "Like most Late Antique men," writes Peter Brown, "Augustine was credulous without necessarily being superstitious," a statement that is amply demonstrated by the accounts of miracles that he included in *The City of God*.[12]

Peter Brown terms Christian asceticism "the *leitmotif* of the religious revolution of Late Antiquity."[13] Not only the abundance of reported miracles but also their ubiquity among all classes of society is striking. Nearly everyone seemed to be personally acquainted with cases of miraculous healing. The greatest preachers, scholars, and theologians of the age were enthusiastic in their acceptance of reputed miracles of healing, including those the modern reader finds lacking in credibility. Athanasius, Ambrose, Jerome (c. 347–419/20), John Chrysostom (c. 347–407), and Augustine believed in the reality of miraculous healing as a contemporary phenomenon and encouraged the dissemination of miracle stories.

Hence one can speak of not only a quantitative but also a qualitative change in this regard when comparing the late fourth century with the previous centuries of Christian history, in which reports of miracles are general, secondhand, and infrequent.

In late antiquity, magic also was used increasingly for healing by Christians and pagans alike. It has been argued that by the late third century the old Roman religious institutions had lost their appeal to all social classes. There was, as a consequence, a spiritual void, which was filled by a variety of new religious manifestations, including the growing influence of magic, which was felt even in the highest intellectual circles. Augustine and other church fathers, however, considered dependence on magical powers and devices reprehensible, because they attributed those powers to demonic forces. For more than three centuries Christians had condemned the use of all magic, including charms and amulets. But in the fourth century the large numbers of nominal converts who entered the church following its legalization in 313 and its growing respectability brought pagan attitudes and practices, such as magic, with them. Augustine complained of Christians who consulted astrologers after finding prayer and natural remedies unsuccessful. Christians commonly adopted the use of amulets, although they may not have viewed them as either magic or specifically pagan. In some cases the church provided alternatives, such as the sign of the cross, which seemed to provide a magic more powerful than amulets.

There is no question that there was a heightened supernaturalism among pagans and Christians alike in the late fourth and fifth centuries. But while some Christian literature of the fourth century, particular saints' lives and apocryphal acts, are indeed marked by an exaggerated supernaturalism, much of it is not. Rational approaches to religion continued to exercise a predominant influence on the thinking of ordinary Christians. Claims of miraculous healing do not account for most of the celebrated conversions to Christianity in the fourth century. Christians did not offer the same promise of healing to pagans that the temple healing of Asclepius could. In spite of the appeal of magical charms and relics in the West, as well as the popularity of ascetics and charms in the Eastern Empire, there appears to have been no diminution in Christians' seeking healing from physicians. The earliest hospitals began to be established by Christians in cities throughout the Eastern Empire at the same time that miraculous claims of healing were making their appeal. Some of these hospitals were staffed by medical attendants. Even ascetics were by no means averse to recommending the use of medicine when they believed it would be efficacious, though they were sparing in using it themselves.[14]

Miraculous healing did not replace Christians' ordinary reliance on medicine. Although it became a highly visible phenomenon in the late fourth century, it was derivative of the ascetic movement. Its source was not ritual healing administered within the context of the liturgy or practice of the church. Rather, it was a highly visible manifestation of divine power that ascetics could exercise and that had not previously been seen in the same way in the church. Rowan Greer views the growing prominence of the saints as setting the stage for the Western Middle Ages.[15]

Medical Philanthropy in the Early Church

From the very beginning, Christianity displayed a marked philanthropic imperative that manifested itself in both personal and corporate concern for those in physical need. In contrast to the pagan classical world, in which no religious impulse for charity took the form of personal concern for those in distress, Christianity regarded charity as motivated by agape, a self-giving love of one's fellow human beings that reflected the incarnational and redemptive love of God in Jesus Christ. At the same time that ordinary Christians were encouraged privately to visit the sick and aid the poor, the early church established some forms of organized assistance.

The administrative structure of the local church (*ecclesia*) was simple but well suited to the supervision of charitable activities that relied on both clerical and lay activity. Each church had a two-tiered ministry made up of priests and deacons, who directed the corporate ministry of the congregation. Deacons, whose main concern was the relief of physical want and suffering, had a special duty to visit the ill and report them to the priests. They received collections of alms every Sunday for those who were sick or in want, which were administered by priests and distributed by deacons. Widows who did not need assistance formed a separate class that later developed into the office of deaconess. They were expected to help the poor, especially women who were sick.

Although their numbers and resources might be small, Christians were equipped, even in the most adverse circumstances, to undertake considerable charitable activity on behalf of those who were ill. Owing to a combination of inner motivation, self-discipline, and effective leadership, in the first two centuries of its existence the local congregation created an organization, unique in the classical world, that effectively and systematically cared for its sick.

In the third century the rapid growth of the church, particularly in the large cities of the Roman Empire, led to the organization of benevolent work on a larger scale. Roman cities were crowded, often unsanitary, and, for large numbers of city dwellers, lonely. Groups such as guilds and burial societies maintained a degree of fellowship and mutual support, but many urban dwellers did not have any family or other social network of support. As the number of those who benefited from the church's charitable activity grew, it became increasingly difficult for the clergy to deal with the demands made on them. Hence congregations began to create minor clerical orders to assist them.

In a letter preserved by Eusebius, written in 251 by Cornelius, bishop of Rome, to Fabius, bishop of Antioch, we learn that the church in Rome supported 46 priests, 7 deacons, 7 subdeacons, and 42 acolytes, as well as 52 exorcists, readers, and doorkeepers—altogether a staff of considerable size.[16] Apparently the church in Rome had divided the city into seven districts, each under a deacon, who was assisted by a subdeacon and six acolytes. They cared for fifteen hundred widows and distressed persons who were supported by the church. Adolf Harnack estimated that the Roman church spent from 500,000 to 1 million sesterces annually on the maintenance of those in need. A century later, John Chrysostom writes that the Great Church in Antioch supported three thousand widows and virgins, along with other sick and poor persons and travelers. All this—the establishment of minor orders to assist priests and deacons, the creation of sizable staffs of clergy in large churches, the regular support of considerable numbers of the poor and sick, and the expenditure of large sums of money—suggests that the churches devoted a good deal of attention to corporate philanthropic activity.[17]

The maintenance of the sick was viewed by the pre-Constantinian churches as part of their charitable ministry. As that ministry grew, so apparently did the number of sick who were supported by the churches. Presumably much of the care was directed toward relieving individual suffering rather than rendering prophylactic or therapeutic treatment, and it is likely that the assistance given was in many cases rudimentary and palliative. The church's care of the sick relied primarily on the clerical orders, which were made up of men chosen for their spiritual rather than their medical qualifications. Their possession of the latter was merely incidental.

In AD 250 a plague spread throughout the Roman Empire that called for a much more extensive effort than churches had previously put forth on behalf of the sick. Commonly called the Plague of Cyprian, it is said to have originated in Ethiopia and spread rapidly through Egypt to North Africa and thence to Italy and the West as far as Scotland, where it reached epidemic proportions. It recurred at intervals in the same district, with brief remissions followed by additional severe attacks. It lasted for fifteen to twenty years and carried off large numbers of the population of the Roman Empire. According to Zosimus, the mortality rate was higher than in any previous epidemic.[18] In some places those who died outnumbered the survivors. In Rome, five thousand people are said to have succumbed in a single day. Except for making supplications to the gods, the civil authorities made little effort to alleviate the situation. Responsibility for health was regarded as a private, not a public, concern. Emergency measures were rarely taken by Roman municipal officials; hence the frequently described scenes in classical literature, from Thucydides to Procopius, of corpses lying unburied in the streets during times of plague.

Without a concept of private charity in classical society, no activity was undertaken by individuals, philanthropic organizations, or temples to ameliorate the condition of the sick during epidemics; they and their families were left to fend for themselves, often with wholly inadequate resources. "Simply put," writes Rodney Stark, "pagan cults were not able to get people to *do* much of anything. . . . And at the bottom of this weakness is the inability of nonexclusive faiths to generate *belonging*."[19] It was the Christian belief in personal and corporate philanthropy as an outworking of Christian concepts of agape and the inherent worth of individuals that introduced the concept of social responsibility in treating epidemic disease.

During the Plague of Cyprian, Christian churches, even though they were undergoing their first empirewide persecution, devised in several cities a program for the systematic care of the sick. In the autumn of 249 the emperor Decius had ordered senior members of the Christian clergy arrested, and a few months later he required everyone in the empire to offer sacrifice to the gods on pain of death. In spite of the constraints of persecution, the bishops provided energetic leadership in organizing the clergy to direct relief efforts for those suffering from the plague. In Alexandria, where the plague reduced the population by more than half in a decade, Dionysius, bishop of the city from 247 to 258, wrote that priests, deacons, and laymen took charge of the treatment of the sick, ignoring the danger to their own lives. As a result, he writes, "the best of our brothers" succumbed to the disease.[20] Their activity contrasted with that of the pagans, who deserted the sick or threw the bodies of the dead out into the streets.

Further evidence of the Christian response comes from Carthage, where Cyprian was bishop. The plague beset the city in 252, causing much havoc. The streets were filled with corpses, which people were afraid to touch. The pagans deserted their dead and dying, while the unscrupulous took advantage of the situation to rob the sick. The Christians were blamed by the pagans for the calamity. This was a common pagan response, as Tertullian's well-known remark illustrates: "If the Tiber floods the town or the Nile fails to flood the fields, if the sky stands still or the earth moves, if famine, if plague, the first reaction is 'Christians to the lion!'"[21] Cyprian responded to the crisis in an address to the Christian community in which he called on Christians to aid their persecutors and to undertake the systematic care of the sick throughout the whole city. He appealed to rich and poor alike for help. The rich gave of their substance, while the poor were called upon for service. He urged that no distinction be made in ministering to Christians and pagans alike. His activity in organizing the care of victims of the plague continued until his exile five years later, in 257.[22]

Although our sources emphasize the voluntary work of the clergy and the laity, it is likely that the ferocity of the plague and the high mortality that it induced forced some churches, perhaps for the first time, to employ burial and medical attendants to assist the clergy. Gregory of Nyssa, describing the same plague in Pontus, says that "more died than survived, and not enough people were left to bury the dead." We can infer from the figures given by Dionysius for Alexandria that the situation there was not much different. According to Dionysius, the Christians undertook the burial of the dead, a task that the pagans refused for fear of contagion.[23] The church had always provided burial for its members, initially as a work of mercy undertaken by fellow members. The burial of victims of the plague may have seemed to Christian leaders a logical extension of the church's duty to the Christian dead. The Christian churches had become so identified with the burial of the dead by the fourth century that Constantine inaugurated free burial services under the direction of the clergy. Julian the Apostate mentioned Christians' concern for proper burial of the dead (along with their hospitality and purity of life) as a factor that had led to the Christianization of the empire.[24]

Although the work of the large urban churches during the plague was done on an ad hoc basis, it probably would not have been so effective had not a system of congregation-centered care of the sick already existed. Indeed, the importance attached to voluntary benevolence by the early church obscures the high degree of organization developed in the pre-Constantinian period. And the genius of the church in adapting itself to the increasing demands for its charitable activities is nowhere more evident than in its concern for the poor and the sick. Even in the earliest stages the church's success in caring for the sick depended as much on the carefully defined duties of its leaders as on lay involvement.

Christian medical philanthropy furnished palliative care, which lay within the ability of those without medical training to provide. But one should not draw the lines too distinctly, since simple therapeutic measures must have been administered when necessary or available. Rodney Stark argues that because there was no concept of social service and community solidarity in the pagan world-view, "when disasters struck, the Christians were better able to cope, and this resulted in *substantially higher rates of survival.*" The palliative care that they offered the sick, even the simple provision of food and water, without skilled medical attention, likely reduced mortality considerably. "Modern medical experts," writes Stark, "believe that conscientious nursing *without any medications* could cut the mortality rate by two-thirds or even more."[25] There was no charitable care of any kind, public or private, apart from Christian diaconal care, because there was no religious, philosophical, or social basis for it. Not only did substantial numbers of Christians survive but since nursing care was given to pagans as well, gratitude may have had an effect on public attitudes toward Christianity. The number of Christiâns appears to have increased during the plague as a result of the decline of traditional social bonds and the creation of new bonds between surviving pagans and Christians, resulting in large numbers of conversions.

The diaconal model of philanthropy was well suited to Christianity's first three centuries, when the urban congregation was the focal point of the movement. It is likely that the great plague of the mid-third century provided the church with its greatest opportunity to extend medical charity. Its ministry to the sick had hitherto been inwardly directed, largely to its own adherents. Increasingly Christian medical care became outwardly focused, now enlarged to include many who were victims of the plague. The administrative structure was already in place. Deacons, aided by those in minor clerical orders, routinely cared for the sick on a large scale, while priests and bishops were experienced in the administration of sizable funds from the collection and distribution of alms. Whether or not bishops made use of a corps of hired medical and burial attendants, their energetic response to the plague marked a significant advance in the church's concept of medical charity. The evidence suggests that for the first time the church conceived of its ministry to the sick as one that included both pagans and Christians, without distinction.

As late as the mid-fourth century, the concept of being a "lover of the poor" (*philoptôchos*) was a novel one in the Greco-Roman world, with no antecedents in classical ideas of philanthropy. Organized care of the poor was contrary to patterns of classical civic beneficence, in which aid was distributed by public benefactors (*euergetai*) to all citizens alike without regard to wealth or status. Within the traditional classical pattern of euergetism (public philanthropy), the rich showed their civic patriotism to the city by sharing their wealth, not just with the poor, but with all their fellow citizens. When the sense of community within the city-states weakened in late antiquity, the old ideological basis for euergetism was replaced by a new ideology of private charity in which one group within society (the poor) was elevated above the rest as recipients of philanthropy.

The introduction of new ideas of almsgiving, which had their origin in Christian rather than Graeco-Roman values, led to a redefinition of the poor. A specific group known as "the poor" (*hoi ptochoi*) had not previously existed in the public eye as long as the community was viewed as a collective whole, one in which all citizens of the city shared in public benefactions. Wealthy pagans continued to espouse the traditional classical view that the poor were passive recipients of fate, and they looked down on them as base and ignoble in character. Christians, influenced by many biblical texts that spoke of the care of the poor as a duty, saw them as especially blessed by God, endued with special grace, and even in their poverty bearing the image of God. They regarded giving to poor as giving to Christ, and philanthropy to the poor as demonstrating love for their Savior. Both donor and recipient came to regard themselves as fellow servants, a theme that one finds repeatedly in contemporary sermons.

Distinctive Christian ideas of charity, which had not enjoyed public recognition until the mid-fourth century, for the first time in classical society both identified and elevated the previously invisible poor as a specific group. Over time, the lower classes of the city, once given a specific identity and defined for the first time as collectively deserving the assistance that had previously belonged to all citizens, would replace all citizens as the beneficiaries of assistance. This little-noticed movement marks one of the truly revolutionary changes in human sentiment in Western history and constitutes a significant feature of the transition from a classical to a Christian society.

The Origin of the Hospital

The principle of the church's duty to care for "the poor" was basic to the founding of the earliest hospitals. The hospital was, in origin and conception, a distinctly Christian institution, rooted in Christian concepts of charity and philanthropy. No pre-Christian institutions in the ancient world served the purpose for which Christian hospitals were created, which was to offer charitable aid to those in need. None of the provisions for health care that existed in classical times and have been suggested as precursors—military and slave infirmaries (*valetudinaria*), temples of Asclepius (*asclepieia*), physicians' clinics (*iatreia*), or public physicians (*archiatri*)—resembled hospitals as they developed in the late fourth century. Roman infirmaries, *valetudinaria*, which were maintained by legions and large slaveholders, have most often been adduced as parallels or precursors, but they offered medical aid to a restricted population (soldiers and slaves) and were never available to the public. Moreover, they were created for economic or military reasons, not as charitable institutions.

Cenobitic, or community, monasticism had from its beginning placed a premium on practical charity of all kinds, particularly medical charity, and the rise of charitable foundations occurred as a result of the growth of the monastic movement. Thus the poorhouse (*ptochotropheion, ptocheion*), which appeared in the early 340s in Constantinople and elsewhere, accepted the sick as well as the poor. In the early 380s, and perhaps as early as the 330s, hostels (*xenones*) that cared for the sick were attached to churches in the capital city. Separate institutions were established for orphans, foundlings, the aged, lepers, and poor travelers. But it was not until the late fourth century that Christian hospitals began to be organized. They were known by a variety of names—*xenodocheia, nosokomeia, xenones*—that came to distinguish them as hospitals that treated the sick.

Andrew Crislip identifies three necessary characteristics of an early hospital: inpatient facilities, professional medical care for patients, and charitable care.[26] All three were found in the best-known and probably the earliest hospital, the Basileias, begun about 369 and completed in about 372 by Basil the Great (c. 330–379), who later became bishop of Caesarea (modern Kayseri), in Cappadocia, Turkey. Basil's idea of creating a hospital (or, as Basil himself termed it, a "poorhouse") had its origins in a famine in 368/69, during which he had organized a distribution of food. His hospital, which he established outside Caesarea, employed a regular live-in medical staff who provided not only Christian aid to the sick but medical care in the tradition of secular Greco-Roman medicine. It included a separate section for each of six groups: the poor, the homeless and strangers, orphans and foundlings, lepers, the aged and infirm, and the sick. The *keluphokomeia* housed lepers, who were gathered together from the countryside around Caesarea into one place where they could be cared for. Gregory of Nazianzus has left us a contemporary, if somewhat idealized, description of the Basileias, in which he contrasts the treatment received by the sick (particularly lepers, the "poor par excellence") with their previous condition. Gregory describes it as

> a new city the treasure-house of godliness . . . in which disease is investigated and sympathy proved. . . . We have no longer to look on the fearful and pitiable sight of men like corpses before death [lepers], with the greater part of their limbs dead, driven from cities, from dwellings, from public places, from water courses. Basil it was more than anyone who persuaded those who are men not to scorn men, nor to dishonor Christ the head of all by their inhumanity towards human beings.[27]

Basil played a pioneering role in establishing the first hospital. As he secured funds for his initiatives, wealthy individuals played an increasing role in establishing hospitals. Municipal bishops long exercised a general supervision of charitable institutions and supported them with ecclesiastical funds. Later they benefited from the largess of emperors.

Hospitals quickly expanded throughout the Eastern Empire in the late fourth and fifth centuries, with bishops taking the initiative in founding them. They spread to the Western Empire a generation after they were created in the East, but owing to economic difficulties their growth in the West was much slower. The earliest Western hospital was established in Rome c. 390 by Fabiola, a remarkable, independent-minded noblewoman who was a friend of Jerome's. Jerome writes, doubtless with some exaggeration, that the hospital in Rome enjoyed such success that within a year after its founding it was known from Parthia to Britain. Fabiola built the hospital with her own funds and worked in it herself, gathering the poor sick from public squares and personally nursing many of them. Her personal participation (like that of Basil's) was a factor that distinguished Christian charity from pagan philanthropy. Hospitals and other charitable institutions were recognized by pagans as peculiarly Christian institutions, and the emperor Julian (r. 360–63) complained that "the impious Galilaeans support not only their own poor but ours as well; everyone can see that our people lack aid from us."[28]

The creation of the hospital marked a major advance in medical care. The Basileias did not, however, immediately replace Christian charitable foundations of a more limited kind, a wide variety of which continued to exist. Monastic orders provided much of the manpower to staff medical institutions. In most cases the model of earlier, palliative care of the sick remained the only care available. Over time some hospitals—always a minority—came to employ physicians. The entry of numbers of Christians into medicine in the late fourth century may have been motivated in part by the desire to serve the ill in hospitals. The first hospitals were founded to provide care for the poor, and it was often terminal care. This too distinguishes it from pagan philanthropy. There were no public or private pagan facilities for the dying, who were prohibited from seeking admittance to the temples of Asclepius, since death within a temple precinct polluted the sacred space. The pattern of the earliest Christian hospitals persisted, and they remained for centuries what they had been intended to be from the beginning, institutions for the indigent, while those who could afford a physician's care received it in their homes.

Chapter Five

The Middle Ages

Since the Renaissance, historians have used the term *Middle Ages* for the roughly nine hundred years between the fall of the Roman Empire in the West in c. AD 500, which marks the end of the ancient world, and the beginning of the early modern period in c. 1400. It has become conventional to divide that larger period into the early Middle Ages (c. 500–c. 1000), which was characterized by anarchy and the disintegration of urban life and Roman civilization, and the late, or High, Middle Ages (c. 1000–c. 1400), which witnessed Europe's resumption of trade with the eastern Mediterranean and the revival of city life, the creation of universities, and the rebirth of classical learning. While these terms, like all historical generalizations, are somewhat misleading, they are useful in framing important periods of transition, of both decline and renewal.

The early Middle Ages were a period of material and cultural change that followed the collapse of the Roman Empire in the West. In the fifth century AD, Germanic tribes made repeated incursions across the Rhine and Danube Rivers and settled within the Western Empire. The Germans were a nomadic, pastoral people who practiced agriculture but achieved greater status from warfare. As desperate peoples seeking havens, they were constantly searching for new lands and shifting their settlements from one place to another. Over time, as a result of their invasions, the Western Empire was divided into independent, largely Germanic kingdoms under native rulers: most of Britain under the Angles, the Saxons, and the Jutes; Gaul (modern France) under the Franks and the Burgundians; Spain under the Visigoths; Pannonia (Hungary) under the Huns; and North Africa under the Vandals.[1] The last Roman emperor in the West, Romulus Augustulus, abdicated in AD 476 and the Ostrogoths under King Theodoric conquered Italy in 493.

The fall of the Roman Empire in Europe and the western Mediterranean led to chaos and disorder on a broad scale. Paved roads, which had been the pride of the Roman Empire, became rutted and in some cases impassable, their bridges washed out. Trade disappeared as society contracted to small isolated communities, while agriculture declined markedly. There was an exodus from urban areas to the country as the system of food supply fell apart. People sought protection from marauding bands of barbarians, and large rural estates replaced cities as centers of population. The origin of castles and noble power lay in the protection they offered in return for labor and services. The structure of government and the rule of law disappeared. Over the centuries, educational institutions ceased to exist, and except for the clergy, society became illiterate. The term *Dark Age* has often been applied to these centuries to denote the wholesale loss of literacy, though historians usually avoid the term today because they believe that the "darkness" of the age is sometimes overstated.[2] Nevertheless, European civilization reached its lowest ebb in the years between c. 500 and c. 1000.

In the midst of shattering military defeats and barbarian incursions, the Christian church was the one institution that both preserved cultural traditions and created islands of structure in the midst of a highly unstable situation. But to speak of "the church" is to misrepresent Christianity's institutional and theological homogeneity in the medieval period. The Western Church, which should be distinguished from the Eastern Church of the Byzantine Empire, encompassed not only cultural distinctions but different liturgical practices, educational backgrounds, theological understandings, and diverse popular and elite traditions. Northern Catholics were markedly different from Italian Catholics, an example that may be multiplied many times. In spite of appearances to the contrary, the church was never a top-down institution in the early Middle Ages.[3] Papal supremacy was always contested, and the ecclesiastical hierarchy concealed much disagreement within the ranks of theologians and the hierarchy itself over major and minor issues. Hence it is unwise to make facile generalizations regarding the medieval church.

Sickness and Healing

The Germanic conquerors brought with them to what had been the Western Roman Empire a folk animism that threatened to overwhelm traditional

Greco-Roman medical approaches to illness. Although Christian missionaries to western and northern Europe tried to eradicate these folk practices, Germanic peoples employed them as alternatives to Christian practices. Some missionaries allowed pagans to continue their older habits as a transitional means to full acceptance of Christian traditions. Gregory I, pope from 590 to 604, wrote in 602 wrote to the missionary Mellitus, who was traveling to Britain, to encourage him to accommodate Christian customs to pagan ones by, for example, allowing the old temples to remain, while destroying their idols and converting the buildings to Christian worship.[4] Animists believed that sacred places were inhabited by spirits, and converting them to Christian churches was more easily accomplished than destroying them. Christian missionaries discovered that Germanic folk medicine included magical incantations and elements of witchcraft, augury, divination, astrology, and sorcery that had been imbedded in Germanic culture for centuries. They also discovered that the Germanic peoples thought these were connected with demons and that they employed them for malevolent purposes.

Examples of pagan practices for healing included placing a child on a roof or in an oven to cure fever or a wife's tasting her husband's blood as a remedy for sickness. Popular too were quasi-medical practices of the kind described in Marcellus of Bordeaux's fifth-century work *De medicamentis* (On remedies), which mingled pharmacology, herbal lore, folk medicine, and spells (both pagan Celtic and Roman in the British Isles) to help individuals treat their own illnesses. Church leaders (but not necessarily laypeople) opposed this magico-medical approach, which often combined spells and incantations with the occult properties of gems and herbs. One sees them repeatedly condemned in conciliar decrees and in handbooks of penance, which listed specific sins requiring confession and repentance and were produced for the assistance of clergy who heard confessions. Missionaries attempted, not always successfully, to substitute specifically Christian formulas such as the Lord's Prayer and the Creed for pagan incantations. In spite of repeated attempts to prohibit pagan healing and other customs that Christians regarded as drawing on preternatural powers, it proved impossible to eliminate them, and they remained widespread throughout the Middle Ages as an aspect of folk culture.

Although many people resorted to folk remedies for healing, a tradition of secular medicine was also transmitted from late classical antiquity to the Middle Ages. Monasteries became the sole repositories of books and learning in the early Middle Ages. Monks were presumed to be literate, but even secular (nonmonastic) clergy ordinarily could not read. Hence learned medicine, which was based on knowledge of medical theory, was limited to monasteries. Monasteries like the abbey of St. Gall, in what is today Switzerland, maintained medical writings in their scriptoria (rooms where monks could read or copy manuscripts).

Already in late antiquity, the philanthropic medicine that hospitals offered was often, perhaps usually, administered by monks, though most were not physicians. As monasteries grew rapidly in number in the early Middle Ages, medicine played an important role in monastic life. Each monastery had an infirmary and an herb garden and collected medical recipes. Many monks began to acquire medical skills informally through apprenticeship or practice. Physicians still provided few truly therapeutic services to the sick. As they had done in classical antiquity, they offered prognosis and diagnosis, while emphasizing prevention over therapy. There were two kinds of physicians, secular practitioners and clerical physicians. The latter were usually monks who had been trained by apprenticeship.[5]

Nearly all who received an education in the early Middle Ages were trained in monasteries and became members of the clergy. They continued to read classical medical literature, for medicine was a part of the curriculum they had studied in monastic schools. Gregory of Tours (c. 540–594) was typical of scholars of the early Middle Ages. He frequently alludes to the sick whose physicians had failed to heal them but who later found healing at the shrine of Saint Martin. He was not, however, opposed to the use of medicine, for he regularly consulted medical and pharmacological handbooks. Gregory found a place in his thinking for both traditional medicine and miraculous healing, as well as for both natural and demonic causality. Medicine and religious healing coexisted without apparent tension, since it seemed evident from the experience of many people that God healed sometimes through natural means and sometimes by religious means.

Greco-Roman medicine in late antiquity was transmitted in a synthesis created by Galen in the second century AD. In late antiquity learned medicine increasingly was acquired largely from books and taught by iatrosophists (medical philosophers). Some Greek medical texts by Galen and Hippocrates were available in the early Middle Ages; they were translated into Latin, since the ability to read Greek had all but disappeared in the West. Early medieval clinical training was probably undertaken exclusively by apprenticeship. It focused on treatment and remedies, with little attention given to physiology or anatomy.

Religious or liturgical healing within the confines of the church, as opposed to healing by ascetics, became securely established in late Roman times. It comprised anointing with oil, baptism, the use of the sign of the cross, and liturgical exorcism. Such practices were found in penitentials, handbooks for clergy who heard confessions. A common feature was exorcism. It is not true, despite frequent statements to the contrary, that demons were widely thought to be the cause of disease. Although forms of mental illness were sometimes attributed to demons in some folk traditions, astrological and humoral explanations were also given in medical literature. The Burgundian Penitential, for example, states that wizards sometimes invoke demons to make men mad. But insanity or "nervous" diseases were just as often explained by natural causes, and physicians invoked medical theories, usually following Galenic theories of humoral imbalance.[6] They also attributed mental illness to other factors, such as overwork or sexual indulgence.[7] Monks who had some familiarity with medical literature sometimes distinguished between natural causes of mental illness and demonically induced states. But they invoked the same naturalistic explanations of melancholia and insanity that were given by medical writers, while at the same time suggesting an additional supernatural influence of demons. The diagnosis often reflected both folk-cultural and medical assumptions based on the same symptoms.

Nevertheless, educated persons in the early Middle Ages, nearly all of whom were clergy, believed in the existence and activity of demons and attributed some diseases to them. Pope Gregory I, one of the best-educated men of his age, encouraged the cult of saints and relics, miraculous healing, and the study of demonology, yet he had a lifelong interest in medicine and retained a personal physician who had been trained in Alexandria. It is difficult for modern readers to appreciate how eclectic medieval people were in their approach to healing. Learned monks and physicians practiced healing sometimes by medical means, sometimes by religious means, and sometimes by employing magic, all within a Christian context. The competition they faced was from pagan folk-magical practices among the Germanic population, who were only superficially Christianized.[8]

During the early Middle Ages monasticism became prominent throughout Europe. Monasticism had begun in Egypt in the third century AD. Monks were men who renounced the world and left society to go into the desert to escape the temptations of wealth, sexual permissiveness, and worldly entertainments in Roman society. They took vows of poverty and chastity. Originally, monasticism was widespread in the eastern Mediterranean, but in the fifth century it was introduced also into the West. Benedict of Nursia (480–543) was one of the founders of Western monasticism. Benedict was born into a noble family, but he gave up his wealth to become a hermit monk. He won so many followers that he organized them into monastic communities in Italy. He composed a Holy Rule that established a pattern of daily life for his monks. Benedict's Rule spread rapidly, and members of his order came to be called Benedictines. Moderate in its ascetic requirements, the Rule was adapted to Western ecclesiastical and cultural practices and maintained high moral standards.

Monasteries flourished during the early Middle Ages in large part because the chaos and destruction of the barbarian invasions led many men to withdraw from a world in ruins to the protection of a sanctuary. They formed ordered communities in the midst of a disordered world. Public opinion venerated them as models of a perfect Christian society, indeed a copy of heaven. Their main purpose was to engage in prayer and worship, but monks performed other work, and they generally did it well. It was by accident that they became preservers of ancient manuscripts. After Benedict's death, Cassiodorus (487–583), a Roman senator, established a monastery in his old age at Vivarium, to which he gave his own large library. After a time, some Benedictine monks began to devote more time to study than they did to manual labor. Each monastery established a scriptorium, where manuscripts were recopied by hand. By encouraging monks to copy and preserve manuscripts, Cassiodorus was indirectly responsible for making monasteries centers of learning. As a consequence, the Benedictines played an important role in the preservation of medical texts.

Monasteries became the thread by which ancient Greek and Roman learning was maintained in Europe for more than five hundred years. The manuscripts that monks copied were not merely from the Bible and the church fathers; they included classical texts of secular books written in Latin as well. Latin was the language of education and scholarship in the Middle Ages. Every educated person in Europe could read and speak it. And the education offered in schools was not only theological but also secular. It consisted of what came to be called the seven liberal arts—Grammar, Dialectic, Rhetoric, Arithmetic, Music, Geometry, and Astronomy—which did not become formally established until the time of Alcuin (c. 735–804) but which were required as a basic education preliminary to the study of medicine. Each monastery also maintained a medical facility for sick monks, and Benedict's Rule admonished monks to care for sick children, guests, and the poor within the confines of the monastery. Cassiodorus too urged his monks who had medical experience to care for the sick: "Learn, therefore, the properties of herbs and perform the compounding of drugs punctiliously; but do not place your hope in herbs and do not trust health to human counsels.

For although the art of medicine is found to be established by the Lord, he who without doubt grants life to men makes them sound." He listed various medical authors whose works he had "stored away in the recesses of our library," including treatises by Hippocrates, Galen, and Dioscorides.[9]

Since there were no schools for medical training in the West, learned medicine, based on knowledge of medical theory, was limited to monasteries. Already in late antiquity the philanthropic medicine that infirmaries in the Latin West offered was usually administered by monks. Some monks acquired medical skills, either formally through learning or informally through practice. Most hospitals began as an outgrowth of monastic medical care. As a result, monasteries became the refuge of the sick and the poor. Some secular clergy acquired knowledge of medicine in order to extend medical care to the poor. Bishop Masona of Merida (Spain), for example, founded a hospital (*xenodochium*) in the sixth century, staffed it with physicians, and sent his clergy out to find patients. In their treatment, they did not distinguish between Christian and Jew, slave and free.[10]

The medical literature that survived from classical antiquity did so because it was hand-copied by monks and kept in monastic libraries. It was extensive and diverse and ranged from general surveys of medical knowledge to treatises that dealt with specific areas of medicine. Some manuscripts contain treatises that deal with medical etiquette and ethics. It is probable that they were composed in an attempt to articulate ideals of character and conduct for medical practitioners, whether clerical or secular. One manuscript that dates from the eighth century exhorts physicians to serve rich and poor alike, looking for eternal rather than material rewards. A manuscript from the ninth century urges the physician to "take care of rich and poor, slave and free equally, or among all such people as medicines are needed." Both enunciate the ideals of Christian medical philanthropy and reflect the compassionate ideal of Christian medicine.[11]

The High Middle Ages

In the eleventh century, Europe began slowly and gradually to emerge from two centuries of attacks by the Vikings, the Arabs, and the Magyars, which had caused even more destruction in Western Europe than had the earlier waves of Germanic tribes that brought about the fall of the Western Empire. The recovery came about through the resumption of trade and commerce, which in turn led to the growth of cities. The source of this revival was the Mediterranean world. During the early Middle Ages Constantinople was the greatest commercial and industrial city in Christendom. But in the seventh century, following the death of Mohammed in 632, Arabs conquered North Africa and spread Islam and the Arabic language throughout the Middle East, North Africa, and the Iberian Peninsula. For the next four hundred years Arab pirates dominated the Mediterranean Sea and almost completely cut off trade between Western Europe and Constantinople. The only European trade with the eastern Mediterranean was a trickle carried on by the Venetians. In the eleventh century these contacts increased as Europeans began to drive the Arabs out of the Mediterranean. Within a century the Arabs had lost all their major ports in the western Mediterranean. And with the beginning of the Crusades in the late eleventh century the port towns of Italy began extensive trade with the Byzantine Empire. The new trade and industry gave an impetus to the rise of towns in Europe.

The first school for medical training in the West was created in the ninth century at Salerno, south of Naples, where a *civitas Hippocratica*, or community of physicians, had settled. The school employed Greek and Latin Christians, as well as Jews and Arabs, as masters. But Salerno was never a single entity or a direct antecedent of the universities. It accepted all students irrespective of nationality, women as well as men. The medical course took five years, and this was followed by a one-year apprenticeship. The graduates practiced medicine throughout Europe.[12] Students had access to a number of short Byzantine Greek medical texts that had been translated into Latin. In the late eleventh century, Constantine the African (c. 1020–c. 1087), a merchant who had become a monk, brought twenty Arabic texts of Galen and Hippocrates to Salerno. He translated them into Latin, first at Salerno and later at the nearby monastery of Monte Cassino, thereby facilitating the transmission of Hippocratic and Galenic medicine into Europe. In doing so he redressed the impoverishment of medical knowledge in the Latin West.

Before Constantine, Latin texts of Arabic works were short and lacked physiological theory. His translations were later adopted in Salerno and in the new universities as the basic texts of the medical curriculum. Constantine created the first comprehensive encyclopedia of medicine in Latin, the *Pantegni*, a rendering of an Arabic text by Majusi, who was known as Haly Abbas in Europe, with ten books each on theory and practice. The *Pantegni* gave the West its first view of Greek medicine as a whole. It was not until the late twelfth century, however, that the majority of Arabic medical texts were translated. Gerard of Cremona, working in Toledo, Spain, translated twenty-one medical works from Arabic into Latin, including the *Canon* of Avicenna (Ibn Sina), which was a standard text in medical faculties until the late seventeenth century. As a result of the translation movement, learned medicine in the Middle Ages became increasingly based on a Greek and Arab tradition.

Between c. 1000 and c. 1200, towns sprang up along trade routes, near harbors, and in secure locations. In short, Europe became reurbanized. Education shifted from rural monasteries to urban cathedrals, which began to replace monasteries in offering advanced education. Cathedral schools developed a broader curriculum than monasteries had been able to offer. The new curriculum included Latin classics from Roman times and some Greek works that had been translated into Latin, since Greek was not taught in European schools. Translation schools in North Africa and Spain produced primarily Latin translations of Greek authors from Arabic texts. They included most of Aristotle's works, Galen's medical works, and Greek mathematical treatises. In the twelfth century a large number of Greek works became available to western Europeans in translation. They were quickly absorbed into the curriculum of the new schools and universities.

About 1200 the first universities began to be established in the prosperous and growing cities of Europe. Between 1200 and 1500 some sixty universities were created. Advanced study was offered in the three higher faculties—theology, medicine, and law—but competence in the liberal arts was a requisite for admission. Medieval universities, the earliest in the world, were founded by the church. In general the approach to medical education was philosophical and centered on texts rather than on empirical investigation. These texts were studied together with commentaries, but in a scholastic manner, employing the methods of logic and dialectic, with definitions being followed by statements of opposing opinion. The style favored speculation rather than empiricism and was entirely divorced from bedside medicine.

In the twelfth century, dissection—of animals, not humans—was reestablished at Salerno. Pigs were usually chosen because of the perceived similarity of their organs to those of humans. Human corpses, which had not been dissected regularly since Hellenistic times, began to be dissected at the end of the thirteenth century.[13] It was during the late Middle Ages that a Galenic system, based on Galenic anatomy and physiology and mediated through Arabic sources and translations, became established in Europe. Not until 1525 were all Galen's surviving works published in Europe. Galenism would last, with modifications during the Renaissance and the sixteenth century, until the seventeenth century and even later.

By the thirteenth and fourteenth centuries the leading medical faculties were the universities of Montpellier, Paris, and Bologna, which provided medical training for large numbers of physicians. The use of the term *doctor* was originally the prerogative of teachers of theology, and medical practitioners appropriated it only gradually after 1300.[14] Learned physicians were often depicted with a book, a urine flask, or a star chart, all of which were symbolic in medieval art of the physician's learning and his ability to diagnose a disease or predict and trace its course, both of which were more certain than the ability to cure. Most people believed that the celestial bodies influenced the natural world, including plant and animal life and the human body. Professing a knowledge of the regularity of the heavenly bodies and an understanding of its implications was important for the learned practitioner's "professional" stance. The linkage between this knowledge and prognosis was an intrinsic part of the Hippocratic legacy. Hence some practitioners considered astrology a useful tool for prognosis.[15]

Given the therapeutic pluralism of the High Middle Ages, there were other healers besides doctors. They included herbalists, midwives, empirics (craftsmen who often specialized in a particular procedure), barbers (who sometimes performed phlebotomy), religious healers, and a variety of folk healers, some of whom were literate, some not. Nearly every village had a "wise woman" (*vetula*) or local healer who had some medical knowledge. She might use traditional herbal remedies mingled with spells and charms that had been passed on for generations. She might also consult physicians and on occasion refer those who had sought her advice to educated doctors. She might even use some of the same procedures that they employed.

Such a woman was Gueraula de Codines, who lived near Barcelona c. 1300.[16] Gueraula was not a physician, though there were female practitioners in the late Middle Ages (while we know of very few from the early Middle Ages). One or two have come to be widely known, such as the abbess Hildegard of Bingen (d. 1179), who was a medical author. A popular medical self-help book, the *De mulierum passionibus* (*On the Diseases of Women*), commonly called the *Trotula*, was written in Latin and later translated into English so that women could diagnose and treat their own diseases. Women were greatly underrepresented in the profession, although midwives and women who offered some form of medical treatment existed in large numbers. They were not limited, as is often thought, to treating females or to obstetrical practice, but they were prohibited from receiving a university medical education, and hence their numbers were necessarily small. Without a medical degree they lacked the requisite knowledge and training that were coming to be expected of learned physicians.[17]

The clergy continued to practice medicine throughout the late Middle Ages. Some priests and monks who had medical training penned medical treatises to help the poor. One of the most famous was the *Thesaurus pauperum* (Treasury of the poor), which listed simple herbs that the poor could gather in the fields. The likely author, Peter Hispanus (Peter the Spaniard), was a philosopher and physician who became pope in 1276 under the name John XXI.[18] Apothecary guilds had a virtual monopoly on drug sales, and Peter sought to provide information to the poor, who could not afford their prices. Teodorico Borgognoni (1205–1296) was another prominent cleric who was a practicing physician. A Dominican friar who studied medicine at Bologna, he became the personal physician to Pope Innocent IV before being appointed a bishop. He continued to practice surgery and wrote the *Cyrurgia* (Surgery), which covered all aspects of surgery in four volumes. Borgognoni introduced several novel surgical practices, including a more antiseptic treatment of wounds, based on his personal observation. The fact that so many priests and monks practiced medicine troubled church authorities, not because they were opposed to medicine but because they feared that the clergy were neglecting their spiritual duties by practicing medicine for the sake of the fees that it brought. Avarice was commonly regarded as a besetting sin of physicians. This popular view of the medical profession brought with it the challenge for physicians of reconciling the expectation of medical charity laid on them with the fees that they charged. This theme is captured in Rogier van der Weyden's painting the *Medici Madonna*, which probably dates from about 1460–64. In the work, which was commissioned by the Medici family in Florence, van der Weyden depicts the Virgin Mary with Child together with Peter, John the Baptist, John the Evangelist, and Cosmas, who was both a patron saint of physicians and protector of the House of Medici. In the painting, Cosmas is shown placing a coin in a handbag that hangs from his belt. According to a legend, Cosmas had accepted a fee for medical treatment that compromised his reputation of not taking fees and illustrated the prejudice that whatever claims doctors might make of their beneficence, they were greedy. This concern led to a canon (ecclesiastical enactment) of the Second Lateran Council, in 1139, that forbade the practice of medicine by regular (monastic) clergy. But it was of little consequence, since it was never incorporated into medieval canon law.

The clergy's role in medicine diminished over time as European society changed from a rural and manor-based society to a more urbanized one (although Europe was still largely composed of agricultural villages), and medicine developed into a secular profession. The growing sense of professionalism among sec-

ular physicians led to the demand for licensure requirements, ostensibly to protect the public against those whom physicians regarded as incompetent medical
practitioners. The first requirements for licensure were promulgated by Roger II
of Sicily in 1140 and strengthened by his grandson Frederick II in 1231. For the
first time in history the practice of medicine was defined as a privilege rather
than a right by the introduction of competency requirements. This was followed
by the organization of medical and surgical guilds by physicians, who wished to
secure and protect their monopoly of medicine and surgical service. By limiting
the practice of medicine to a group who could establish their competence, the
medical profession could claim to be acting in the public interest.

As an authoritative international body in an age in which governments were
weak, the church routinely extended its jurisdiction over medical guilds by granting charters and enforcing them. Because the church was often involved in granting and protecting medical or surgical guild monopolies, it was able and, from a
medieval perspective, obliged to exercise coercive jurisdiction over areas of life
that would now be the concern of either secular authorities or professional organizations. So, for example, medical and surgical corporations often attempted
to prevent unlicensed persons from practicing by pursuing them in ecclesiastical courts, where the penalty could result in excommunication. Authorities also
sometimes attempted through a variety of means to prevent Christians from obtaining medical or surgical services from Jews or Muslims, the concern being the
potential for spiritual harm. The spiritual obligations of the physician to patients
were of central importance to ecclesiastical authorities, since the care of the
soul was even more important than the care of the body. Nevertheless, because
of a continued shortage of graduates of the medical faculties, Jewish physicians
were sometimes allowed to practice, though they were expelled from England
and France in the thirteenth century. Occasionally, because of their skills, they
reached the highest levels of society, including royal and papal courts. In Italy
civic physicians (*medici condotti*) were also hired to ensure that each city would
have a competent medical practitioner. And some clergy sought and received
dispensations from the church's prohibition against practicing medicine.

The medieval church was concerned with the moral implications of various
occupations, which were addressed in the confessional literature termed *summae confessorum*. These *summae* were intended as tools to aid the clergy in the
interrogation of penitents by providing the priest who heard confessions with
questions designed to uncover and deal with specific professions. One occupa-
tion they addressed was that of medical practitioner. Several *summae* stressed the

responsibility not to practice medicine unless the practitioner was competent. One *summa* asserted that physicians' expertise must be judged according to accepted standards and that simply having a degree was not sufficient.

Practicing without the necessary competence, even if one was licensed, was a sin. If a physician harmed a patient from ignorance, whether by omission or commission, he sinned. Harming a patient by negligence was also defined as a sin, as was experimenting on patients, particularly on the poor or religious (monks or nuns). Keeping abreast of medical literature and techniques was a physician's responsibility, as was consulting with colleagues when in doubt. Rash treatment was condemned. Physicians in doubt about the effects of a particular medicine should leave the patient in God's hands rather than expose him or her to the danger of an untried medicine. Surgeons in doubt about the need for an operation or about their own ability to perform it should leave the patient in God's hands. The physician sinned who intentionally failed to administer an effective medicine that cured quickly merely in order to prolong the illness and collect additional fees. These provisions became enshrined in codes of professional ethics, which lasted until modern times. In the medieval world, which lacked such professional codes, these strictures were given moral force by the church.

Hospitals

In describing medieval hospitals one's definition is crucial. In the Middle Ages, as in early Christian *xenodochia*, hospitals were intended, not for those with acute conditions, but for those, chiefly the poor, who suffered from chronic conditions or old age and were unable to care for themselves. In many instances they were places in which to die. Those in the Latin West were more like hospices, while the largest of the Byzantine hospitals emphasized secular medicine. The sick who could afford care saw physicians in their homes. Most monasteries had long had their own infirmaries, where sick monks could be treated by fellow monks, some of whom might be doctors. Benedict, in his Rule, had established specific directions for the treatment of monks who were ill, and they remained in force in Benedictine monasteries. Over time many monastic infirmaries admitted laypeople to their facilities, which were, however, without the implications of institutionalization that the term *hospital* implies in our own day.[19]

In Western Europe in the early Middle Ages, monastic hospitals were rural, as was society at large. Some hospitals had beds for just a few patients. The treatment they administered was usually not medical but palliative. They offered shelter, food, and care, which the poor lacked. Even minimal care could be, and often was, curative. Many hospitals did not admit those with contagious diseases, for fear of their spreading infection. Caregivers recognized that a healthy soul contributed to the health of the body, and one writer has described the care that medieval hospitals offered as psychosomatic medicine.[20] While those who administered care were aware of the importance of rest, diet, and nursing care, they recognized that the "passions of the soul" were important in healing, and they especially encouraged cheerfulness. Basil had considered psalmody important in nourishing the soul, and music played an important restorative role in hospitals in the Latin West.

Many of the best-known hospitals in later Europe date from medieval times. The Hôtel-Dieu in Paris was founded, according to legend, in 651; St. Bartholomew's (Barts) in London, in 1123; and St. Thomas's in London, in 1170. In the tradition of Christus medicus, administering spiritual medicine was the first duty of medieval hospitals. "Receive the patients as you would Christ himself," read the rule of the Hôtel-Dieu. "Treat each patient as if he were the master of the place." All three hospitals continue to operate today, but in vastly different circumstances from those of their earliest life.

Unlike hospitals in the Byzantine Empire, most hospitals in the Latin West did not have physicians. The monks and nuns who cared for the patients might, however, have considerable medical knowledge, acquired by devoting their lives to the care of the sick. Beginning in the eleventh century, or in some cases earlier, many of these hospitals offered medical as opposed to merely palliative care, and they increased the number of patients they cared for.

Patronage was important in the foundation of hospitals. Wealthy patrons or nobles often would found a hospital in return for the monks' saying perpetual prayers for their souls. Hospitals were founded as well by merchants or guilds, though they were invariably staffed by monks and nuns. They differed from early Christian hospitals in their size, some of them being quite large. Santa Maria Nuova, in Florence, was founded in 1288 with only twelve beds for the sick and poor (it served as both a hospital and a poorhouse). It could hold 250 patients in 1500, by which time it took in only the poor who were sick. It was admitting some 3,000 male and an additional number of female patients annually, with a cure rate (according to its records) of more than 80 percent. Its first practitioners, a physician and a surgeon, were hired by 1350, and by 1500 it boasted ten doctors in residence, a pharmacist, and additional assistants.

The success of Santa Maria and other Italian hospitals in large cities in northern Italy, such as Florence, Siena, and Milan, by the time of the Renaissance can be attributed in great part to the wealth of those cities.[21] So famous did Santa Maria become that when Henry VII of England looked for a model for the hospital he proposed to build (the Savoy, which was constructed between 1505 and 1517), he requested that Florence send him the statutes of Santa Maria. From 1300 to 1500 the number of hospitals devoted to the care of the sick grew rapidly. By 1428 there were 35 hospitals in Florence alone. There were 400 in England, and the number had increased to 750 by the time of the Reformation. Paris had 12 hospitals, as well as a lazar house (a place of confinement for lepers or those with infectious diseases) and an asylum for the blind, in the thirteenth century. Most hospitals consisted of huge halls divided by partitions. They were usually supervised by Augustinian monks and nuns, who formed the best-known nursing orders (both St. Bartholomew's and St. Thomas's in London were at one time Augustinian houses). The nursing care was performed by lay brothers and sisters who were members of a religious order but performed manual labor, though many hospitals were overcrowded and dirty, and the care was sometimes poor.

Leprosy and the Black Death

Of all diseases that afflicted Europeans in the Middle Ages, leprosy was the most terrifying. *Leprosy* was a generic term for many skin diseases that became common in Europe from the end of the eleventh century to the fifteenth century, with the growth in the numbers of lepers paralleling the growth of cities.[22] Because of the instinctive revulsion that many felt for lepers, they were rigorously excluded from the community. More than any other disease, leprosy was considered symbolic of the disease of the soul. The physical symptoms were popularly regarded, though not by physicians, as an outward manifestation of internal spiritual corruption. This fear occasioned much legislation to cordon lepers off from all outsiders. Yet the incidence was not high, probably no more than four or five per one thousand.

At the same time that the leper experienced the fear of society and its ostracism, he or she could also represent the image of Christ, who in the Incarnation had taken on human flesh and had suffered in order to redeem the human race. Such was the physical and spiritual ambiguity of leprosy that it was believed that God visited lepers more intimately than others. In the late medieval period private philanthropists, rather than municipal authorities, founded leprosaria called lazar houses, or lazarettos, in which lepers were housed and served by nonlepers (though the earliest in the Latin West was founded in sixth-century Gaul). Lazarettos were named for Lazarus, of Jesus's parable (Lk. 16:19–31), who was thought to have been a leper, reflecting the medieval belief that lepers were especially favored by God. The purpose of their confinement was to protect society from contagion. Because it was popularly believed that leprosy was a divine punishment for sexual immorality, lepers were often required to take a vow of chastity in order not to transmit the disease to others.

The greatest plague of all time in the Western world was the Black Death, which initially erupted in Messenia, Sicily, in 1347 and lasted until 1351, and then returned periodically during the next four centuries. The Black Death was so called because of the dark skin blotches that were symptomatic of the disease, which was a variety of *bubonic plague*, a term that did not arise until long after the fourteenth century. The plague had long been endemic in parts of Central Asia, and we know that it existed in the ancient world; it is probably the disease mentioned in 1 Samuel 5–6. In the sixth century AD, during the reign of Justinian (r. 527–65), it broke out first in Egypt in 541 and lasted for fifty years in the Mediterranean world.

The bubonic plague is primarily a disease of rats; it was carried by black rats and spread by their fleas to human beings. There are three forms of plague: bubonic, pneumonic, and septicemic. The actual plague bacillus was the *Yersinia pestis*, which was not discovered until 1894.[23] Its most characteristic symptom was the appearance of buboes, or swellings of the lymph nodes. The black swellings, which were about the size of an egg or a small apple, appeared in the armpits and the groin. They oozed blood and pus and were followed by spreading boils and black blotches on the skin from internal bleeding. The sick suffered severe pain and died quickly, usually within five days of the first symptoms. As the disease spread, a second form, with other symptoms—continuous fever and spitting of blood—appeared in place of the buboes. Victims coughed and sweated heavily and died even more quickly, within three days or less and sometimes within twenty-four hours. In both types the fluids that issued from the body smelled foul, adding to the loathsomeness of the disease.

No known epidemic disease in human history has been as devastating, with mortality rates from 30 percent to 50 percent in the first four years. That of Florence was much higher, while Milan was spared. New public-health measures were adopted, including the quarantine, first introduced in 1377, and the designation of lazarettos, which were meant to isolate and provision the sick poor. Physicians gave medical and astrological reasons for the plague, the most common being the corruption of the air, and they recommended both prophylactic measures and conventional medical treatment.[24]

Popular explanations abounded, many of them of a moral nature, but they should not be taken for those of learned physicians. There was, however, no antagonism between those who sought religious origins of the plague and those who suggested natural ones. Nevertheless, because of the extent of the plague, it was widely believed to represent divine retribution for human sins. Avarice and usury were the most commonly alleged sins. The most frequent religious responses included offering intercessory prayers and making processions. Sufferers sought the aid of plague saints, such as Saints Sebastian and Roche, as well as Job and the physician saints Cosmas and Damian.

A few Europeans were driven to bizarre religious practices. Some joined the Flagellants, who believed that they could be purged of their sins and hence escape God's punishment by flogging themselves with leather whips that were studded with iron spikes. They marched from city to city, stripped to the waist, crying aloud to God to spare them. They put on regular performances three times a day. Women accompanied the Flagellants in a separate section, as the latter interceded with God for humanity. Others walked in religious processions barefoot and dressed in sackcloth, sprinkled with ashes, weeping, pulling at their hair, carrying candles and relics, sometimes with ropes around their necks. Still others took refuge in Satanism, in mystical cults, or in a dancing mania such as St. Vitus's dance. There grew a morbid fascination with the grotesque, the revolting, and the necrophilic. Treatises on the art of dying (*ars moriendi*) became immensely popular, as people believed that death was imminent and they should prepare for it. In some cases, Jews or lepers were persecuted. They formed a convenient minority that could be readily demonized, since they were already unpopular for economic and social reasons. Communities of Jews were sometimes attacked by mobs who blamed them for the epidemic and burned hundreds to death as scapegoats. These extreme manifestations of popular hysteria, however, constituted a small minority of religious responses.

The Black Death produced a wrenching break in the continuity of life in Europe. The plague was so devastating that it did not inspire in people the desire to help those who had contracted it. This was a common reaction in time of plague. Instead of helping, many were inclined to flee, since flight appeared to be the only recourse with which to escape death. Even family connections were hard to maintain. Some fathers abandoned their wives to escape infection, and some wives left their children. Members of two professions, priests and physicians, faced a crisis of conscience. The plague was so contagious that priests or doctors who visited the sick exposed themselves to the likelihood that they would contract the disease and die. Many fled, but records indicate that at least half of them stayed to do their duty.[25] The result was that their numbers suffered disproportionately from death. Even then the church lost prestige and spiritual authority because it was widely perceived to have failed people during their sufferings. As a result, anticlerical feeling grew. Moreover, the experience of suffering seems not to have bettered the spiritual or moral condition of many people. Some contemporary observers thought that the moral state of society was worse after the plague, with people more avaricious, more bellicose, and more litigious. The plague last appeared in northern Europe in the 1660s and in Marseilles in 1720, after which it largely disappeared, though a reappearance of epidemics caused it to be reported in several countries at the end of the twentieth century.[26]

Relics and Pilgrimages

Among Christians the veneration of relics (the remains of a holy person, generally bones or dust, as well as objects that had contact with his or her body) can be traced to the Christian martyr Polycarp, who died in c. AD 155 and whose tomb became a pilgrimage site. Christians collected and preserved relics of martyrs in late antiquity and sometimes celebrated the Eucharist at their tombs. The cult of relics spread quickly in the West and became popular in the early Middle Ages among all classes of Christians. The appeal of relics and the miracles associated with them was widely used in missionary efforts to convert the Germans, who were not drawn to theological subtleties but found hope and comfort in relics that had been associated with saints. More than any other factor, it was the sense of the miraculous that appealed to the barbarians who overwhelmed the Latin West. While the medieval church offered a variety of kinds of Christian healing, including prayer and anointing with oil, none of them came close in popularity to relics. In the eighth century, the practice arose of making pilgrimages a form of penance. This, together with the growing veneration of Christian saints, led large numbers of medieval Christians to seek healing by means of relics. The belief that healing came through direct contact with relics, most often by touching them or sleeping next to a tomb, necessitated a pilgrimage to the site where the relics were preserved. Those who suffered from acute diseases and thus could not stand the long journey or afford it tended to consult local practitioners.[27]

In the central Middle Ages the doctrine of the treasury of merits, which was proposed in the thirteenth century and formalized in the fourteenth, permitted the granting of an indulgence for the performance of good deeds as penance. The indulgence gave access to the infinite merits of Christ and the saints. The doctrine of penance was abused when clergy promised a decrease of suffering in purgatory. The extension of penance to pilgrimages provided an impetus to the practice of traveling, sometimes long distances, to pilgrimage centers. During the Crusades (1095–1295) the practice increased enormously, with large numbers of pilgrims making the long and dangerous trip from western Europe to the Holy Land. Before the arrival of the Crusaders an order of volunteers was formed in Jerusalem to care for sick pilgrims. They organized themselves according to the rules of the Benedictine order and took monastic vows, adopting the Maltese cross as their symbol. They became known as the Knights of the Order of the Hospital of St. John of Jerusalem—or Hospitalers—after the Crusaders conquered Jerusalem in 1099.

The Hospitalers were divided into two classes, the "brothers infirmarians," who administered a hostel in Jerusalem, and the "military brothers," who policed the routes that pilgrims took to the Holy Land. The latter eventually developed into an army that garrisoned castles and fought battles. Later, a third class, of chaplains, was added to minister to the spiritual needs of the order. Under their first known administrator, Master Gerard, they received papal approval in 1113, coming under the direct administration of the pope and exempt from lay or ecclesiastical jurisdiction. The hospital they created in Jerusalem served between nine hundred and one thousand patients, who were segregated by sex into eleven wards. The Hospitalers made no distinction between Christian, Jewish, and Muslim patients except to respect the dietary restrictions of each faith. Like most early hospitals, theirs maintained what we would today regard as a small staff, in this case four physicians. The statutes of the order gave instructions on "How our Lords the Sick should be received and served." They required that large beds be provided for the patients, each one having its own sheets and covers. Diet played an important role in care, with bread made of special fine flour. On Saladin's capture of the city in 1187, the order was forced to move from Jerusalem, and it eventually built a new hospital in Acre. When Acre fell in 1291, the Hospitalers went first to Cyprus, then to Rhodes, which they controlled for some two hundred years, devoting themselves during that time increasingly to military functions. But they also built small hospitals in Europe, beginning with a hospital in Montpellier founded by Augustinians that they modeled on the hospital in Jerusalem. This was followed in 1204 by a hospital in Rome that was dedicated to the Holy Spirit. Augustinians subsequently founded Holy Spirit hospitals throughout western Europe.

The increase in trade with the eastern Mediterranean during the Crusades and the demand for relics led to a profitable traffic in objects that had been ostensibly associated with saints, members of the holy family, or martyrs. Relics were required for the consecration of a new church, and they came commonly to be used as amulets. Many educated and uneducated Christians believed that they possessed supernatural power, particularly to heal disease and restore health. Churches found it profitable to possess relics, for which they might create a shrine that would attract pilgrims. Reliquaries that once housed relics can still be seen in every major and many minor Catholic churches and sacristies in Europe.

Three of the most desirable pilgrimage sites were Jerusalem, Rome, and Santiago de Compostela, the last associated with the traditional burial site of the apostle James in northwestern Spain. Along its famous pilgrimage route were established hospices, hostels, and shops of cobblers, barbers, and other merchants who could meet the needs of pilgrims after each day's journey. Pilgrimages became the theme of story and legend. Chaucer's *Canterbury Tales* describes a disparate group of pilgrims as they travel to the shrine of Thomas Becket at Canterbury. While the vast majority of pilgrims undertook a pilgrimage as penance, many sought healing, more often from "popular" (uncanonized) saints than from "official" (canonized) ones. According to Ronald Finucane, 90 percent of the miracles that we find recorded at European shrines were miracles of healing. As with instances of religious healing at pilgrimage centers of other ages (e.g., that of the god Asclepius in Greece and Rome), stories of miraculous healings circulated and gave encouragement to those who had come seeking relief. But accounts of miracles were not merely anecdotal. Those who were associated with maintaining shrines kept meticulous records. They reveal few instances of healing of epidemic or acute infections. Congenital and chronic diseases were the most common, as in antiquity. Those who experienced healing included cripples and paralytics (about 50%); the deaf, mute, and blind (15%–20%); and those who were mad or possessed by demons (10%).[28]

Not all healings were instantaneous, nor were they necessarily permanent or complete. One hesitates to apply modern concepts anachronistically to healings at medieval pilgrimage sites, and it is unhistorical to assume only modern rationalistic categories, but it seems natural to assume that some of them were psychogenic or brought about by permanent or temporary remission (e.g., in such diseases as arthritis or asthmatic conditions). In cases of relapse, pilgrims might return to the original source of healing. At some pilgrimage centers, clergy, who had limited knowledge of medicine but access to a good monastic library of medical works, were available to treat those who came with a medical problem. But

such was the demand for relics that pious frauds, as well as traffic in relics and reports of counterfeit miracles by dishonest priests, abounded. So widespread did
the manufacture of fraudulent relics become that Erasmus famously remarked
that there were enough pieces of the true cross to build a battleship.

The Byzantine Empire

In AD 330 the emperor Constantine transferred the capital of the Roman Empire from Rome to Byzantium, an ancient Greek city on the Bosporus at the entrance to the Black Sea, which he renamed Constantinople (City of Constantine).
He and his successors ruled over a united empire until 395, when on the death of
the emperor Theodosius the Roman Empire was divided between his two sons.
The two halves were never reunited. Between 395 and 493 the Western Empire
fell into swift decline, while the Eastern Empire (which came to be known as the
Byzantine Empire), possessing more secure boundaries and a more prosperous
economy, remained in existence until it was captured by the Ottoman Turks in
1453. Although it had been refounded by Latin-speaking Romans under Constantine, Constantinople was always a Greek city. The population spoke Greek, and
they inherited the rich cultural traditions of classical and Hellenistic Greece.
While much of Roman civilization in the West would be destroyed by barbarian invaders, Greek educational institutions, libraries, and scholarship remained
strong in the East, where the standard of living was higher.

The Eastern, or Orthodox, Church, as it came to be known, was ruled by the
patriarch of Constantinople, but in practice the emperor had effective control
over the church in a system that became known as Caesaropapism. Over time
the Eastern Church assumed a very different character from that of the Western
Church, which owed its allegiance to the bishop of Rome, who acquired the title of pope. The fortunes of the Eastern Church followed those of the Byzantine
Empire. Originally very powerful and benefiting from a close alliance with the
Byzantine emperors, it enjoyed the patronage of the state and built thousands of
churches in Asia Minor, Syria-Palestine, and other parts of its large empire. Orthodox theology, which was complex and subtle, its particular liturgical practices, and
a mysticism rooted in monastic life permeated the culture and the world-view of
Byzantine society, which was markedly different from that of Western Europeans.

Byzantine Hospitals

The origins of the earliest hospitals should be seen against the backdrop of
social, economic, demographic, and religious factors that emerged in the east-

ern Mediterranean in the fourth century AD. Drought and famine drove large numbers of people from the land and into the cities, leading to a social crisis in eastern cities that had not existed earlier. The earliest hospitals were created in the Eastern Empire, beginning with Basil's celebrated Basileias in Caesarea, in Asia Minor. The Arian controversy (the dispute over the nature of Christ and whether he was God or a created being), which seriously divided Eastern Christianity, may have played a part in the creation of the hospital. Some scholars believe that Basil borrowed his ideas from Eustathius of Pontus, a semi-Arian bishop. The creation of Byzantine hospitals (*xenones* and *nosokomeia*) grew out of the concept of *philanthropia* (love of mankind), which was a basic theme in Orthodox theology. The Greek term *philanthropia* was used in the Hellenistic period by the wealthy and by rulers who condescendingly shared their wealth with those beneath them. But Greek Christians adopted the term to reflect the idea of agape, the love of God for humankind that was seen in the incarnation of God in Christ. It was found particularly in Byzantine monasteries and would be claimed as an attribute by Byzantine emperors, who maintained a reputation for *eleemosyne* (almsgiving). *Philanthropia* provided the ideological basis of benevolence and charity, whether of bishops, private philanthropists, or emperors.

Bishops had from the beginning played a prominent role in the foundation of hospitals, and they long continued to exercise a general supervision of charitable institutions. But over time wealthy individuals would play an increasing role in establishing hospitals, and they of course demanded some control over them. The emperors too showed great interest in hospitals, to which they granted gifts and exemptions from taxation. They were responsible for the largest foundations, such as the Pantokrator, which was founded in Constantinople as part of the monastery of Christ Savior Pantokrator in the twelfth century. It hired physicians and five pharmacists. Five wards contained fifty beds in all, divided according to the diseases diagnosed. A female physician (*iatraina*) treated women in a separate ward. An outpatient clinic was staffed by two surgeons and two physicians. Many Byzantine hospitals were monastic foundations, which spread rapidly throughout the Byzantine Empire, thanks to gifts from the emperor, wealthy patrons, and bishops. Others were independent or under patriarchal control.

Another factor was the spread of cenobitic monasticism and the premium that it placed on charity of all kinds, especially medical philanthropy. Virtually every hospital established in the earliest period (370–451) was founded by monks. But not all monastic orders sought to practice Christian charity through medicine. A major question that was much disputed in Orthodox monasticism concerned the relationship of *theoria* (the contemplative life) to *praxis* (acts of mercy and benevolence). The tension between those who advocated participation in the world through active philanthropy and those who sought withdrawal from it to pursue a life of prayer was never resolved, and it affected the operations of Byzantine hospitals for centuries.[29]

Basil's hospital became the model for institutions throughout the Eastern Empire. The Byzantine hospital accepted all classes, not only the poor. There was a wide range of specialized early Christian charitable institutions, not all of which cared for the sick. Constantinople had an orphanage (*orphanotropheion*), as well as institutions that served the poor (*ptocheia*), the homeless (*xenones*), and the aged (*gerokomeia*). All were under the patronage of the emperor. Only a minority of the *xenodocheia* had the resources to employ physicians. Peregrine Horden estimates that in the pre-1204 period from twenty-three to twenty-five Byzantine hospitals had physicians. Some maintained, in addition to bed, board, and nursing care, permanent medical attendants and trained assistants. Those most commonly employed were *hypourgoi*, assistants with no particular medical training. It would be an anachronism to speak of a professional hospital "staff." But it is for the most part in Byzantine hospitals that one finds staff physicians at all; in Western Europe, except in Italy, there were few physicians in hospitals until the end of the Middle Ages.[30]

Within the Byzantine Empire, physicians trained at the Alexandrian school in Egypt, where medicine was still being taught until the Arab conquest in the seventh century. They took a course that lasted for about four years and was based on sixteen of Galen's major works. Greek medical treatises from the classical and Hellenistic periods were readily available and could be read by physicians in their own language. In addition to encyclopedic summaries by Oribasios (c. 325–c. 400) and Aetius of Amida (fl. c. 500), which included passages from works by Galen and other Hellenistic and Roman physicians, physicians used the works of Paul of Aegina (fl. late seventh century) and Alexander of Tralles (fl. sixth century). In Constantinople, physicians undertook apprenticeships at hospitals as well as in schools operated by the church. Delivery of infants was left to midwives. Lepers were not permitted in ordinary hospitals but were treated in specialized institutions.

Spoudaioi and *Philoponoi*

Not as well known as the hospitals for which Byzantium became famous were the lay orders of *spoudaioi* and *philoponoi*, found in the cities of the Eastern

Roman Empire in late antiquity and the Byzantine period. The spoudaioi were "the zealous ones"; in Egypt they were known as philoponoi, "lovers of labor." They were attached to large churches in the great cities of the East—Alexandria, Antioch, Constantinople, Beirut, and Jerusalem, most prominently—although they are attested for smaller cities as well. The spoudaioi comprised both laymen and laywomen who adopted ascetic practices that included chastity (or continence for those who were married) and fasting. Their functions varied somewhat according to local traditions, but in most cities their ministry was twofold: to care for the sick and to perform liturgical functions, such as reading scripture, chanting, praying, and participating in funerals, vigils, and processions. While they represented a branch of the ascetic movement, they never constituted a monastic order. Although laypersons, they came to be recognized as an intermediate order between the clergy and the laity, and they are so described by several sources. We find frequent mention of them from the fourth through the seventh centuries and a few scattered references thereafter.[31]

Our sources indicate that a chief function of the spoudaioi was to provide assistance to the indigent sick of the urban areas in which they lived. One finds descriptions in the sermons of late antiquity of the poor and disabled that congregated in public places—a woman lying in labor in a church portico at midnight; the poor seeking warmth in the public baths on winter nights. This kind of poverty had long existed in the Mediterranean world. What was new was that it was noticed by Christians, who saw the homeless poor as a discrete group who needed assistance. It was to the urban poor, sick or dying on the streets, that the spoudaioi devoted their service. The spoudaioi would search the streets and alleys by night for those who were ill, distribute money to them, and take them to the public baths. Although they were medical attendants, they had no medical training. The functions they performed, moreover, were those that would ordinarily be performed only by members of the lowest classes.

There is no evidence to associate either order with hospitals. Hospitals arose independently of the spoudaioi and were based on different principles. They did not seek out patients, and they offered medical care when resources permitted. In Alexandria, members of the lay order of philoponoi carried the sick from public places to the church of SS John and Cyrus, not to a hospital. They presumably employed ad hoc arrangements approximating those used in time of plague to house the sick.

Hospitals and the lay orders coexisted as complementary models of the church's care of the sick. The lay orders provided services beyond those the hospital could offer: They actively sought out the urban poor who were scattered in public places and who might find access to hospitals difficult. They flourished where there were large churches to sustain them. These orders simply carried on the practice long established in Christian churches of offering the kind of assistance to the sick that deacons and deaconesses could perform.

Religious Healing

From late antiquity, ascetics gained great influence in the Eastern Roman Empire and became a marked feature of Byzantine life. Known to offer miraculous healing, they were sought out by the sick who could not find healing from physicians or who suffered from chronic diseases. While their importance in healing has been overemphasized (they were not as ubiquitous as some scholars imply), there is no doubt that they became local patrons and benefactors who carried great influence with those in positions of authority. They became the subjects of hagiographic literature, which records their many miracles and exorcisms, the latter performed by anointing with oil, prayer, making the sign of the cross, or touching the afflicted with the clothing of a holy person. But they healed only a minority, perhaps a very small minority, of those who needed healing. And they sometimes worked with local doctors, to whom they would on occasion refer a particular case. Moreover, there was antipathy between physicians and shrines of healing. If healing by ascetics was free, it was not cheap: they required the sick who sought their healing to confess their sins and do penance.

The great churches of Byzantium became healing centers that were associated with their possession of sacred relics, which were kept in reliquaries. As in the West, there was much trafficking of relics. Churches' desire to have them led to a trade in the bones of saints and articles associated with them. Several churches claimed to have the skull of John the Baptist. Painted icons later became known for their healing potency. The best-known shrines were those of Cosmas and Damian, legendary twin brothers who practiced medicine without accepting payment and were therefore known as *anargyroi* (lit., "silverless [moneyless] ones"). They were martyred c. 285, and because they were famed for their miracles of healing, many churches were dedicated to them. They were frequently portrayed in art, sometimes shown holding a medical bag or a chest of medical instruments.

Some saints specialized in healing particular diseases. Thus Saint Photeine could cure blindness; Saint John Prodromous, hernia and diseases of the genitals; and Saint Febronia, women's diseases. Perhaps no saint was more popular as a healer than Saint Artemios, who specialized in healing hernias and diseases of the testicles and genitals and whose relics were in the church of Saint John Prodromous.[32]

Healing at the shrine of a saint might be sought by buying a votive candle or by obtaining consecrated oil or holy water from a sacred spring. The most interesting method of religious healing, however, was incubation, sleeping in the aisle or the portico of a church or near a tomb with the expectation that a healing saint would appear in a dream. It became popular for serious medical conditions in the sixth century and continued to be used throughout the entire Byzantine period. Incubation had been the most common form of pagan religious healing in the classical world, where it was sought by pilgrims in the sanctuaries of healing gods such as Asclepius and Serapis. It went back even further, to the pharaonic period of Egypt, and it continues in Greek churches to the present day. No practice better illustrates the cultural continuity of healing practices across religious and national boundaries.

Magic was widely used in the Byzantine period, as it had been in late Roman times. It extended to the highest classes. Amulets (*phylakteria*) were small tokens that one carried in one's pocket or wore around the neck. Each token bore the image of a saint or an invocation suited to a particular disorder. Women carried amulets during their pregnancy to guarantee the safe delivery of the child they were carrying. The medical writer Alexander of Tralles (fl. sixth century) occasionally prescribed amulets for colic because some patients would not follow their prescribed regimen or take their drugs.[33] Christian authorities condemned sorcery, as they had during the Roman Empire, since they believed that it owed its efficacy to demonic powers. But condemnation did not prevent amulets from being used extensively. Many of them incorporated traditional symbols, such as geometric shapes, lunar crescents, and serpents. They were inscribed on lead tablets or on tiny rolls of papyrus that could be placed in amulets or worn around the neck. Wearers sought protection against a variety of perceived threats, especially demons. Also readily available were curse tablets, which called down diseases or death on their enemies. A common use of magic was to protect ritual books of magical spells that contained incantations for the prevention or treatment of illnesses or protection for childbirth against demons who could cause miscarriage. Astrological medicine also enjoyed respect in the Byzantine Empire, as it did in the West.

Chapter Six

Islam in the Middle Ages

with Mahdieh Tavakol

Islam is a monotheistic religion that was founded by the Prophet Muhammad, who was born in AD 570 in Mecca, Arabia, and died in 632 in Medina. The religion of Islam is based on the belief in the oneness of God (Allah), in God's revelation to his messengers and prophets, and in the resurrection and the afterlife. The basic beliefs and principles of Islam are articulated in the Quran, the sacred scripture, and by the teachings and normative example (Sunnah) of Muhammad, who is believed by Muslims to be the last messenger of God. The Quran was allegedly revealed to Muhammad over a period of twenty-three years and is considered by Muslims to contain the verbatim word of God. Muhammad did not claim to have created a new religion but introduced Islam as the continuation and completion of a primordial divine message that God had revealed to earlier prophets, including Adam, Noah, Abraham, Moses, and Jesus, in different periods of human history.

The Quran and the Sunnah, which include both acts and sayings of the Prophet Muhammad (known as Hadīth), have been the main sources defining the Islamic world-view and providing a comprehensive rule for human conduct. The Quran contains the main articles of the Islamic faith and general instructions applicable to social and individual aspects of life. As an application of these instructions to behavior, manners, and thought, the Sunnah of the Prophet Muhammad has been regarded by Muslims as a source of guidance regarding issues that were not regulated in detail in the Quran.[1]

By the end of Muhammad's life the whole Arabian Peninsula had come under the flag of Islam. Arabian tribes and city dwellers either converted to Islam or, in the case of Jews, Christians, and Zoroastrians, were permitted to practice their faith while paying the tax designated for non-Muslims. When Muhammad died, there was a dispute in the nascent Islamic community about who should succeed him. Two tendencies were expressed: one, which would become the Shia interpretation of Islam, favored the continuation of Muhammad's religious and political authority under the leadership of his cousin and son-in-law 'Alī ibn Abī Tālib; the other, which constituted the majority and would become the Sunni interpretation, favored the leadership of Abū Bakr (r. 632–34), who actually became the first caliph.[2] Four caliphs—Abū Bakr, 'Umar, 'Uthmān, and 'Ali—who ruled from 632 to 661 as successors of Muhammad, are known as the "rightly guided caliphs" (*al-rāshidūn*).

A bitter civil war led to divisions in the Muslim community, particularly for the control of the caliphate, and resulted in the domination of the Umayyad Dynasty, which ruled over the Islamic world from 661 to 750. In less than a century, Arab conquests extended Islamic rule from Spain in the West to northern India in the East, creating an empire that was larger than the Roman Empire at its peak. Arabic, the language of the Quran, became the common language of religion, literature, and administration, as well as the spoken language of much (but not all) of the Arab conquest. In the mid-eighth century, the Abbasid Dynasty (750–1258) replaced the Umayyads. Under the Abbasids, who made Baghdad their capital, Islamic civilization flourished, and several branches of the arts and sciences, including architecture, astronomy, mathematics, optics, and medicine, developed. This period of prosperity and cultural growth is sometimes referred to as the Islamic golden age.

The relationship between Islam and medicine can be viewed in two different ways. In a conceptual approach, we can see how medical concepts such as health, illness, and therapy are introduced by the main Islamic sources (the Quran and the Hadīth). In a historical approach, we can see how Islamic beliefs have influenced the development of medical knowledge and practice among Muslims. We will first concentrate on the conceptual framework of Islam as it relates to the definitions of health, illness, and cure. Then we will address the historical developments of learned medicine and the establishment of hospitals in medieval Islam, as well as the influence of religion on those developments. Finally, we will describe the various modes of actual medical practice in traditional Islamic society and their relation to religion.

Islamic Concepts of Health and Illness

In the Islamic world-view, the human being is considered to be God's representative and viceregent on earth, created in the best possible form and with the best divine instructions for the purpose of knowing and worshiping God and returning to him. Only healthy human beings can fulfill their religious obligations fully and accomplish the purpose of their creation, although those who are sick also have religious and ethical obligations. A Muslim is obliged to care for his or her body as a religious duty and expected to be concerned with its health, since the body is not simply a private human possession but rather a gift entrusted to one by God.[3] The belief that a human being is not the real owner of his or her body, but only its owner in this life, has obliged Muslims to treat it appropriately. Islam views health as God's hidden blessing to his people, a blessing whose value can be better sensed and appreciated when it is absent. Muslims are advised to appreciate this blessing by carefully preserving health and showing thankfulness to God, who has bestowed it. Petitions for health are a common part of normal prayers for Muslims whether they are in good or ill health.

The concept of health in Islamic sources is not limited to physical wellness but refers to a holistic concept that embraces physical, mental, and spiritual well-being. The word *illness* (*marad*) is used in the Quran both literally and metaphorically. In the first sense, it means any bodily disorder or malfunction associated with physical pain and suffering. In its metaphorical sense, on the other hand, *illness* can refer to diseases of the soul and the spirit, such as disbelief, hypocrisy, jealousy, lack of piety, and doubt about the existence of God. While illness in its metaphorical sense is associated with divine admonition and damnation, physical illness is connected with God's mercy and comfort. This compassionate attitude toward the sick is expressed in Quranic verses that exempt the ill from religious obligations such as fasting, pilgrimage, ritual washings, and some social obligations. Hence the sick do not need to feel inferior to others or guilty toward God if they cannot fulfill their religious or social duties.[4]

Among Muslims, one common explanation for disease and illness is that illness is a gift of grace and an opportunity to become purified and have one's sins forgiven by God. In another teaching in the Quran illness is a divine test. The Quran depicts the world as a trial in which the believer is occasionally tested in his faith by the Creator: "He has created death as well as life, so that He might put you to a test [and thus show] which of you is best in conduct, and [make you realize that] He alone is almighty, truly forgiving." According to the Quran, God created the world with all its beauties and wonders, pains and sufferings, and he tests his people: "We test you [all] through the bad and the good [things of life] by way of trial; and unto Us you all must return." Therefore, any joy and sorrow in this world, including illness and suffering, can be a test of faith, patience, and trust in God. The story of the prophet Job, who persevered in his faith and remained patient and thankful to God in the time of severe hardship, illness, and suffering is an example of God's test of his prophet portrayed in the Quran.

Illness is viewed as a test not only for the ill but also for their relatives and friends in dealing with the ill and caring for them. The sickness of parents, for example, is considered to be a divine trial for their children, who are advised to care for their parents and treat them with the utmost respect and compassion.[5] In Islam, illness is not something to be hated or despised; as a test of faith and trust in God, it can have chastening, expiatory, and even meritorious effects. The view that illness and ultimately death are divine punishment for sin is emphasized less in Islam than in Christianity.[6]

The Islamic Understanding of Cure and Therapy

Like *marad*, the word *shifā* (healing, recovery, cure, therapy) is used primarily metaphorically in the Quran. In this sense the Quran itself is often mentioned as a source of healing for spiritual illnesses. In one specific reference to physical illness in the Quran, Abraham describes his God to unbelievers as he "who has created me and is the One who guides me, and is the One who gives me to eat and to drink, and when I fall ill, is the One who restores me to health."[7]

With regard to physical disease, Islam obliges its followers to treat their illnesses and restore their health by using medication. Although particular medical cures are not generally referred to in the Quran, there are a few exceptions. In one verse, honey is mentioned as a cure for human diseases. "[And lo!] there issues from within these [bees] a fluid of many hues, wherein there is health for man. In all this, behold, there is a message indeed for people who think!" (Quran 16:69). Emphasizing that God had sent down a medicine for every illness, Muhammad advised believers to use medication to treat their diseases. But how could referring to medication for cure be consistent with trust in God and belief in him as the sole agent of healing? In Islam, God is seen as the first cause of healing, and it was he who bestowed curative powers on medical substances.

The therapeutic measures are only the means through which God's healing takes place. Muslims are supposed to apply the natural means that God created for healing, while at the same time being aware that the healing effect of medical cures depends on God's will and that the realization of a cure can only take place with his knowledge and permission. This belief is reflected in a story about Moses, who while he was ill refused to use the medication offered to him because he believed that God knew about his illness and could cure him without medication if he willed it. But God warned him about his attitude, emphasizing that he wanted his people to seek healing through the means he had created. In this sense, using medication is in reality nothing other than turning to God.

Based on these teachings, there has been no serious opposition to medical treatment among Muslims. One sees occasionally a case such as that of the famous Sufi woman of the eighth century, Rābi'ah al-Adawiyya, who refused not only to use medication but even to pray to God for her recovery, asking, "Who has willed illness—is it not God?" This attitude, however, was not widespread and was even opposed by the vast majority of Sufis, who believed in healing and medical treatment.[8]

Medicine in the Early Islamic Period (610–750)

Before the emergence of Islam in Arabia in the first third of the seventh century, Arabs had a tradition of medicine that consisted for the most part of magical rituals and amulets but also of empirical medicine that included the use of certain seeds and herbs, such as cumin and caraway; animal products, such as the gall of the wolf and camel's milk and urine; and surgical practices, such as cupping and cauterization. Underlying these empirical and folk-medical measures was a deep-seated animism, in which illness was attributed to the intervention of forces exerted by animate entities, such as the genie or the evil eye. The genie, as a spirit present in the physical world, was believed to be responsible for epidemic diseases, madness, and diseases of children, while the evil eye, as a malevolent force, was considered responsible for accidental injuries. Even though these beliefs and practices were challenged by the introduction of Islam, folk modes of medical practice persisted in Islamic lands, particularly in the rural areas. It was only with the gradual theological development of Islam from its original form to a highly articulated religion in the seventh and eighth centuries that the animistic parts of traditional popular medicine came to be regarded increasingly as unacceptable.[9]

At the time of Muhammad there were in Arabia a few medical men who were somewhat familiar with Greek medicine, the best-known among them being al-Hārith ibn Kaladah (d. 670). Despite early contacts with medical schools of foreign origin, however, Muslim Arabs did not seriously practice medicine during the first century and a half after the time of Muhammad. The most notable physicians of this period were Christians, Jews, and sometimes Zoroastrians, who, having received their training in Greek or Persian medicine, worked mostly for the members of the upper middle class in courts in urban areas.[10]

Physicians usually received their training through either apprenticeship or personal tutoring. The majority of Muslims, however, adopted a popular medicine whose concepts and medical recommendations were derived from basic Islamic sources. This popular medicine covered a range of recommendations regarding personal hygiene, dietary restrictions, and folk therapeutic measures. An influential source of popular medical recommendations was collected in prophetic medical books, which greatly influenced Muslims' daily life and later gave rise to a medical genre called "prophetic medicine" (*al-tibb al-nabawī*), discussed later in this chapter.

The Translation Movement (750–900)

In the late eighth century, after Arabic had become the lingua franca of the Islamic world, Muslims who came in contact with other civilizations actively studied their intellectual resources and translated into Arabic the major works of classical Greek, Persian, and Indian sources. The Abbasid ruler al-Ma'mūn (813–833) founded a translation center, the House of Wisdom (Bayt al-Hikmah) in Baghdad, where translation activity reached its peak. The intense translation work, which continued for more than two centuries, made accessible in Arabic the works of Aristotle, Plato, Hippocrates, Ptolemy, and Galen, among many others.

Despite its non-Islamic origin and orientation, Greek medicine was warmly received by Muslims and rarely encountered hostility even in religious quarters. Still, a few jurists, experts in Islamic law, rejected Galen and other Greek medical authorities and supported some kind of prophetic medicine instead. To be sure, considering the religious sensitivities of the Muslim reader, translation from Greek into Arabic came with modifications. Translators usually removed polytheistic elements from Greek medicine, for example, and replaced references to Greek gods (such as the invocation of Apollo, Asclepius, and Hygieia in the Hippocratic Oath) by references to God. In a medical context, these alterations made the medical texts more acceptable to the monotheistic reader, even though the Muslim audience knew that ancient Greeks were not monotheistic and that they worshiped various gods and goddesses.[11] Hence the translation program was not a passive process in which every famous foreign source, regardless of its content, was translated into Arabic. Translation was a selective process that actively determined the role that foreign cultures would play in shaping Islamic culture by deciding which specific works to translate and by making adjustments to troublesome passages and interpreting everything according to Islam.

The Rise of Islamic Medicine (900–1300)

Simultaneously with the translation movement, Muslim scholars started to assimilate and enhance this new knowledge. Over the next several centuries they created an advanced medical corpus. While in the first fifty or so years the translation movement mostly consisted in rendering existing Greek medical knowledge into Arabic, the later phase (from c. 900 onward) was devoted to forming a new medical tradition that included conducting original medical research and writing independent medical treatises and compendia based on the integration of the Greek, Persian, and Indian traditions into an Islamic perspective.[12] With the serious engagement of Muslim scholars in the development of medical knowledge, the medical profession, which originally had been drawn to Christian, Jewish, or Zoroastrian medicine, became totally Muslimized. As a result, Muslims created a major medical tradition that would later influence Western medicine.

Among the physicians who became prominent during this period were Rhazes (Muhammad ibn Zakariyyā Rāzī, 865–925) and Avicenna (Abū 'Alī al-Husayn ibn 'Abd Allāh ibn Sīnā, c. 980–1037). Rhazes was a polymath and a prominent Persian physician who directed a major hospital in Baghdad in the early tenth century. It is reported that to determine where to build the hospital, Rhazes hung pieces of meat in different places in the city and examined them after a few days; he built the hospital where the meat had been least infected. Among many other contributions, he was the first to differentiate between measles and smallpox and to describe the distillation of alcohol and its use in medicine. Although he studied and wrote on different philosophical and scientific subjects of his time, he was most talented in medicine and composed medical works of particular importance. His books on medicine, especially *al-Kitāb al-hāwī*, translated into Latin under the title *Liber Continens*, came to be regarded as classics and were extensively used by later authors.

The Muslim scholar Avicenna, who was both a philosopher and a physician, also contributed greatly to medical science. He was a brilliant student in different branches of learning and wrote on various subjects. His medical compendium *al-Qānūn fi-al-tibb* came to be known as *The Canon of Medicine* after it was translated into Latin in the twelfth century. It was a standard medical text at many European universities until at least the end of the sixteenth century.[13]

The reasons for the reception and assimilation of Greek medicine by Muslim scholars, which resulted in the subsequent rise of learned medicine in Islamic lands, were linked to the development of rational and intellectual schools in Islam, on the one hand, and to its appreciation of medicine as knowledge that could be applied to the benefit of human beings, on the other. Moreover, in line with Islamic teachings about the value of human life and the preservation of health, medicine was granted a special place because of its service to humans, who were viewed as God's representatives on earth. Some Muslim scholars even considered the study and practice of medicine to be a "common religious duty" (*fard kifayah*),[14] a major obligation to God that, if some people fulfilled it, would relieve others from having to do so. The high status accorded to medical knowledge and practice in Islam encouraged Muslims to pursue medicine and develop their medical knowledge.

Greek medicine appealed to Muslims because of the consistency between its underlying philosophy and a basic Islamic emphasis on balance and harmony. The principle of harmony of natures and humors in Greek medicine made it easily digestible to Muslims, who believed in a harmonious universe within which a life of balance and moderation should be maintained. Islamic teachings also influenced Muslims' attitude toward learning pharmacology, anatomy, and physiology. Muslim physicians were encouraged to pursue pharmacology to find cures for diseases because, according to the prophetic sayings, for every disease God had sent a cure. Almost all major Islamic medical encyclopedias, such as Avicenna's *Canon*, have sections devoted to pharmacology.

The study of anatomy was also viewed as valuable knowledge in the Islamic context, inviting Muslims to contemplate nature and their own existence as pointers to God's wisdom and power: "And on earth there are signs [of God's existence, visible] to all who are endowed with inner certainty, just as [there are signs thereof] within your own selves: can you not, then, see?" Muslims viewed the study of the human body not only as a crucial part of medical knowledge but also, as Galen had famously written, as a way to understand God's wisdom in his supreme creation. Nevertheless, Muslims' anatomical and physiological knowledge relied heavily on Galenic anatomy and physiology, as Shari'ah, the religious law of Islam, which was derived from the main Islamic sources, did not permit the dissection of the human body. Human dissection was viewed in Islam as a violation of the human body, which was to be respected as God's most noble creation. Nonetheless, there was no consensus among Muslim jurists on the prohibition of dissection.[15]

The Development of Hospitals

While several sources of medical treatment, such as barbershops and shops selling herbs, including herbal remedies, existed in medieval Islamic society, the public bath enjoyed primacy. The traditional public bath was built originally to provide facilities for performing the ablution rituals required by Islamic law. Gradually it also became an important center for primary health and hygienic services. All segments of society availed themselves of steam baths with hot and cold air and water, massage, and the services offered by barbers and bloodletters. Both traditional and learned physicians prescribed baths for various therapeutic purposes.

As for hospitals, during the lifetime of Muhammad there were no hospitals in Arabia. Under the Umayyad Caliphate (661–750), several houses were built that offered care to the blind and lepers, but they could hardly be called hospitals. The first regular hospital established by Muslims was founded in Baghdad under the Abbasid Dynasty, in the early ninth century. Soon after, similar institutions were built in Baghdad and other important cities, such as Damascus and Cairo, and hospitals gradually spread throughout the Islamic world. While they were open to people from all social classes, and some villagers would go to nearby cities for treatment, they were generally centered in urban areas, to which the rural population had little access. In addition to building urban hospitals, governments developed plans to send itinerant doctors to remote areas and to establish mobile hospitals in rural locations where potential patients did not have access to physicians. Evidence is lacking, however, to indicate whether such plans were implemented and, if so, how successful their implementation was.[16]

Several religious incentives contributed to the foundation of Islamic hospitals. One was the close connection in Islam between faith and good deeds as requirements for salvation. According to the Quran, "those who attain to faith and do righteous deeds" are destined for happiness and for paradise. Another incentive was the importance of community in Islam and the need to maintain tight bonds among its members. A large number of prophetic sayings encouraged Muslims to practice good will toward others, particularly those within the Muslim community. "Muslims are like members of one body," reads one. "If one member is hurt and feels pain, the whole body feels pain." "A person cannot have faith if he satiates himself while his neighbor goes without food," reads another.

A third incentive was the emphasis placed on personal charity. In the Quran, charity is an essential element of piety. "[But as for you, O believers,] never shall you attain to true piety unless you spend on others out of what you cherish yourselves; and whatever you spend—verily, God has full knowledge thereof." Charity will be rewarded by God. "The parable of those who spend their possessions for the sake of God is that of a grain out of which grow seven ears, in every ear a hundred grains: for God grants manifold increase unto whom He wills; and God is infinite, all-knowing."[17]

The emphasis on charity as a meritorious act that brought a divine reward motivated Muslims to contribute to the development of hospitals and pharmacies, which people generally supported through charitable trusts or an endowment (*waqf*). Donations in the name of a *waqf*, according to Shari'ah, usually consisted of different kinds of property, such as agricultural goods, shops, mills, caravanserais, or even entire villages. The revenues from properties endowed for medical purposes were allocated for building and maintaining hospitals and also sometimes for providing small stipends to poor patients upon their dismissal from a hospital.

An Islamic hospital usually served several functions. It might serve, for example, as "a center of medical treatment, a convalescent home for those recovering from illness or accidents, an insane asylum, a retirement home giving basic maintenance needs for the aged and infirm who lacked a family to care for them, and a venue for medical education."[18] To be sure, not all these functions were offered in every Islamic hospital in the Middle Ages. But some of them offered wider services than their Christian counterparts. The allocation of a special ward to the care of the insane, for example, was unprecedented and was taken seriously by Muslims even in the establishment of their early hospitals. Moreover, despite the emphasis on ethical and religious beliefs that required a physician to believe in God and observe his laws, medical practice in Islamic hospitals was generally secular.

After Greek, Persian, and Indian medical sources began to be translated into Arabic in the eighth century, Islamic hospitals were staffed by physicians trained in Galenic, Persian, or Indian medicine. Medical practice was based on the principles of humoral pathology, without the involvement of religious rituals. At least from the tenth century on, Muslim, Jewish, Christian, and even pagan doctors worked together in hospitals and treated patients regardless of their race or religion. This climate of high religious tolerance, however, did not exist to the same degree everywhere, and friction and intercommunal tensions did sometimes arise.[19]

Learned Physicians and Islamic Medical Ethics

With the development of medical and philosophical knowledge among Muslims, the figure of the *hakīm* (lit., "wise person," "sage") emerged in Islamic society. The hakim, who was often at once a physician and a philosopher and was responsible for the improvement of both body and soul, enjoyed a high status in Islamic society. Many prominent Muslim philosophers, such as Avicenna and Averroës (Abū l-Walīd Muhammad ibn Ahmad ibn Rushd, 1126–1198), were also accomplished physicians who made their living by practicing medicine. In addition to scientific competence, medical skills, virtue, and moderation in all areas of life, which Greek medical ethics also demanded of physicians, the hakim was expected to have a firm belief in God, his prophets, and his laws. The Muslim physician viewed God as the ultimate source of healing—in Islam one of the names of God is Shafi, "the Healer"—and saw himself as the instrument for the execution of God's will.[20] In this context, the intellectual and practical powers of the hakim were expected to be intimately tied to his religious faith and reliance on God.

In spite of common positions with Greek medical ethics on some ethical matters, such as the duties of medical practitioners, the ethical code of medical practice in the Islamic Middle Ages cannot be described as merely reproducing Hippocratic ethics, since Islamic medical ethics also incorporated specific Islamic elements. With its emphasis on prevention of disease, Islamic medicine aimed at preserving and restoring health and was not concerned with the enhancement of physical appearance. In other words, while a healthy body was considered to be desirable for the spiritual journey of the soul in this world toward God, the Greek ideal of the beautiful body was notably absent from Islamic medicine. Furthermore, because Islamic society held a very different set of values from those of Greece, Muslim physicians were not supposed to seek, as Hippocratic physicians did, "good repute among all men for all times" for their service. Rather, they hoped for reward from God in this life and in the life to come. The Muslim doctor was responsible to God for his deeds, and his moral failure was viewed as demonstrating a lack of faith and piety. For example, a doctor who performed an abortion that was not medically necessary, which was forbidden by Islamic law, was responsible before God for his wrongdoing.

The Islamic emphasis on equal treatment of friends and enemies, the rich and the poor, and citizens and slaves alike also was hardly compatible with the ideals of Greek society. With an altruistic attitude shaped by the religious emphasis on help and mercy toward the needy, physicians were supposed to treat sick persons gently and to supply their needs more quickly than their own. In contrast to Hippocratic ethics, which discouraged doctors from treating chronically ill patients who were overmastered by their disease, Islamic medical ethics prohibited refusal to treat patients by physicians, whose very presence could alleviate the suffering of the afflicted, even though the physician might not be able to cure them.[21] These ethical precepts were ideals set for physicians who practiced medicine in Islamic societies but who, needless to say, did not always honor them.

Popular Medicine and Islamic Moral Conduct

Although in the medieval period medicine flourished and hospitals were built throughout the Islamic world, learned medicine based on Greek humoral pathology was not the only method of medical practice or even the dominant one. Learned medical practice was usually sought in serious cases and was mostly accessible in urban areas. In less serious cases and with regard to daily matters of health, the majority of Muslims used a popular medicine that was rooted in their religion.

Islam provided believers with a set of medical recommendations and a guide to proper medical conduct. The behavioral teachings of Islam were expressed in the form of divine laws or prophetic recommendations, the keeping of which was viewed as the natural outgrowth of Islamic belief. In fact, their inclusion in the Islamic catalog of commandments guaranteed their application by observant Muslims. These teachings covered a broad range of rules and recommendations, including those related to medical care, personal and social hygiene, dietary habits, medical ethics, and occasional medical advice.

Among these teachings, Islam's emphasis on cleanliness and personal hygiene as a sign of faith strongly influenced Muslims' personal behavior in relation to health. Brushing one's teeth, especially before reading the Quran, was highly recommended, and ritual cleanliness required Muslims to wash themselves regularly, particularly before worship and prayer. While cleanliness was a required condition for worship, outward cleanliness was viewed as a prelude to inward and spiritual purification.[22]

Islamic dietary injunctions also affected Muslims' attitude toward health. Dietary restrictions, which included not only total abstention from alcohol and pork but also fasting, eating less than one had an appetite for, eating slowly, and many other recommendations, were directly or indirectly related to health and medicine. While medication for curing disease and restoring health was recommended and even obliged in some cases, not every kind of remedy was permitted. A remedy could be employed only if it did not contain substances prohibited by Islamic law, such as alcohol and pork.[23] The Islamic emphasis on moderation as a key principle of conduct was to regulate behavior of observant Muslims in all aspects of life including diet. The wasteful use of anything (*isrāf*), including excessive eating and drinking, was opposed as a sin (Quran 7:31), while moderation and adherence to Islamic law were viewed as keys to health and long life. In addition to these recommendations for personal conduct, there was behavioral advice for treating others while they were sick. Visiting the sick was highly recommended in Islamic teaching as a moral duty, and the visitor was described as a person who walked toward the heavens until he returned from the visit. The visit was supposed to be brief, and the visitor was encouraged to take a gift for the patient and to offer hope and encouragement.

Prophetic Medicine

Collections of prophetic medical advice have greatly influenced Muslims' daily life and gave rise to the medical genre called "prophetic medicine." The written source of prophetic medicine was basically compilations by later Muslim jurists of sayings on matters of health and illness that were attributed to the Prophet. The first treatises were compiled in the eighth and ninth centuries, while the compilation of separate books on the subject has continued throughout later Islamic history. Although many of these teachings may transmit genuine sayings of the Prophet, over the centuries collections also incorporated elements of Arabian folk medicine and Galenic medical knowledge. Prophetic medicine is prescriptive rather than descriptive. It emphasizes preserving health and preventing illness by "leading a well-regulated life, following a moderate diet, and avoiding the familiar sources of illness or injury." In addition to recommendations and advice for personal hygiene, proper dietary habits, and the properties of some substances and foods, collections of prophetic medicine include healing techniques such as cupping, bloodletting, and occasionally cautery. Regardless of their application or avoidance of other kinds of medicine, almost all Muslims were familiar with prophetic medicine and followed its recommendations.[24]

As some historians of Islamic medical tradition have indicated, advocates of prophetic medicine apparently wanted, on the one hand, to have a medicine that was separate from a "secular knowledge" of non-Islamic origins and, on the other hand, to defend the practice of healing against those who opposed the application of any kind of therapy. They viewed Galenic medicine as inferior to prophetic medicine in the same way that they considered folk medicine to be inferior to Galenic medicine. Lawrence Conrad, however, does not accept the view that prophetic medicine was a product of Muslim opposition to Greek medicine. He argues that it was a logical and natural result of an interest in medical matters among a religiously educated public, which was familiar with collections of prophetic sayings that had sections devoted to medical and health issues. Conrad believes not only that Greek medicine was not criticized in collections of prophetic medicine but that it permeates these collections. He observes that Plato, Aristotle, Galen, and Hippocrates were occasionally mentioned as medical authorities in those collections.[25]

Miraculous Healing

The miraculous healing performed by Muslim mystics, or Sufis, is another form of cure that has been present in Islamic society. The Quran, unlike the Old Testament, omits any mention of miraculous healing except for the healing narratives of the leper, the blind, and the raising of the dead, all attributed to Jesus by the Quran. The Prophet Muhammad was never introduced in the Quran as a paradigmatic healer, as was Jesus. The Prophet's everyday behavior in matters of health, however, became a normative guide for Muslims, whereas Jesus, whose life was filled with various miracles, never played a similar role in the lives of Christians.[26]

Despite the absence of an emphasis on miraculous healing in Islamic belief, Sufism and the healing practices associated with it developed at least a century after the emergence of Islam. Early Muslim mystics began to adopt ascetic practices, such as seclusion, celibacy, poverty, and charitable work. They usually acted as moral leaders and persuasive preachers, arbiters in disputes, and social critics in society, and fantastic deeds, such as miraculous healing, also were often attributed to them. Sufism became highly developed in later Islamic history. Muslim saints were ordered in hierarchies headed by the highest spiritual guide (*qutb*) of the age. The miracles attributed to a Sufi saint were considered proof of his spiritual power. These miracles included the ability to read minds, to appear in different places at the same time, and to become invisible. The Sufi could also command different creatures, such as predatory animals. He could miraculously bestow food on the hungry, comfort on the distressed, and fertility on the barren, while a common miracle of a saint was to heal the sick and relieve his pain.

Not only was the saint himself venerated but his tomb came to be venerated as a center where people sought grace, blessing, and healing. Despite opposition to Sufism, pilgrimage to the tombs of saints became increasingly popular. The purpose of a pilgrimage might be a simple desire for a blessing and spiritual support, or it might be healing of a serious illness. In the latter case, specific parts of the shrine might be allocated for the sick to sleep in, as in the ancient practice of incubation. The sick person expected to be cured or sometimes to receive instructions for healing in a dream. On some occasions the sick took rags or other objects, such as oil or water, from the shrine because they thought these objects possessed a healing effect.[27] Like doctors, saints could have different specializations, such as healing the blind or the leper or even exorcising demons and curing mental illnesses. Popular Islamic literature refers to Sufi healing saints as common figures of everyday life. However, it is not possible to judge how prevalent the claims of miraculous healing have been in Islamic society. One reason might be that Muslim mystics, unlike Christian saints, were expected to conceal their miracles.

Magical Practices

Throughout Islamic society, while religious recommendations relating to health and hygiene, as well as the teachings of prophetic medicine, were more or less interwoven into everyday life, various forms of medical practice that included astrology, magical healing, and miraculous healing coexisted alongside learned medicine. The pre-Islamic magical beliefs of Arabia blended with the spiritual and magical beliefs of other peoples with whom Muslims came into contact in the course of their territorial conquests, and they provided the basis for magical medical practices. Despite the opposition of Islamic teaching to magic, magical healing was practiced. Also the use of amulets survived among people of different levels of society, although this practice took on a religious appearance. Writings on amulets and talismans came to be limited often to quotations of verses from the Quran instead of magical symbols and words prevalent in the magical practices of pre-Islamic Arabia. For Muslims, magical invocations were most often, although not exclusively, addressed to God rather than to demons, and they served as supplications for God's support and protection against epidemics, the evil eye, and assorted devils and demons.[28] And to some extent, astrological belief and reliance on specific properties of minerals and gems became integral parts of medical practice, whether folk or learned.

Persisting Themes

From an Islamic perspective, the body is a divine gift whose care is obligatory for Muslims. While health is seen as a blessing from God, illness is considered a divine test for one's faith, patience, and trust in God, as well as an opportunity for the physician and other Muslims to demonstrate their concern for the ill. Besides the meritorious effects of a successfully passed divine test, illness could have expiatory and chastening results. Muslims see God as the primary and ultimate source of cure and therapy, since he has provided for human beings medical substances with healing powers. God also heals directly when he wills. Muslims are, however, obliged to refer cases of sickness to physicians and to use medication as the means through which God's healing takes place.

Historically, the pursuit of medical knowledge and practice, as well as the development of hospitals, enjoyed a high status in Islamic culture owing to the emphasis Islam placed on serving human beings as God's representatives on earth. Through translating the major medical works of ancient authors, most importantly Greek authors, Muslims became active in the assimilation and enhancement of medical knowledge. As a result, Islamic culture produced many prominent physicians and created a rich medical tradition. Although the practice of learned medicine and Islamic hospitals were not religious in the exclusive sense of the term, both were influenced in their development by Islamic law, theology, and world-views in general.

Despite the development of learned medicine in medieval Islam, many Muslims adopted a popular medicine that was interwoven with their religious beliefs. The Quran and the prophetic traditions (Sunnah) of Muhammad, as the two basic sources of Islamic belief, not only shaped Muslims' understanding of health and illness but also provided them with a popular medical framework that included recommendations for physicians, patients, and society at large. Islamic popular medicine was generally a preventive medicine that emphasized the preservation of health by leading a well regulated life, following a moderate diet, and avoiding the causes of illness. Among the most important sources that influenced the content of popular medicine in Islamic lands were the collections of prophetic medicine, which covered a broad range of recommendations regarding personal health and hygiene and occasionally included medical treatments. Miraculous healing and magical medicine also coexisted with learned and popular medicine in Islamic society, while magical medical practices were modified to make them more consistent with Islamic beliefs.

Many of the medical practices described in this chapter were prevalent in the Islamic world until the nineteenth century, when they were gradually replaced by modern Western medicine. Even though many Muslims embraced modern medicine, the older tradition of Islamic medicine has survived to some extent in Muslim lands, and there are signs here and there of its revival today. Even today, the popular medicine described in this chapter shapes the way many people view medical concepts and treatments from a religious perspective.

Chapter Seven

The Early Modern Period

When Martin Luther (1483–1546) nailed his Ninety-five Theses to the door of the castle church at Wittenberg, he inaugurated not merely a schism from the Catholic Church and a new branch of Christianity that came to be called Protestantism but a very different way of conceiving of man's relationship with God. Four separate traditions arose out of the Protestant Reformation: Lutheran, Reformed (Presbyterian), Anabaptist (Baptist, Mennonite), and Anglican (Episcopal). They were united largely by their basic differences with Rome but by no means constituted a uniform movement.[1]

The Protestant Reformation provided an intellectual and structural framework that encouraged transitions in a variety of fields, including medicine. Martin Luther introduced the doctrines of *sola fide* and *sola gratia*. Luther rejected the late medieval Catholic assumption that one's meritorious deeds can contribute anything to one's justification. He equated Christian faith with trust in God's promise of salvation and taught that this salvation occurs in a dramatic moment of conversion from reliance on one's good works to earn God's favor to trusting that Christ's sacrifice alone was completely sufficient for one's salvation. For Luther, salvation was a free gift from God. Some Protestants, such as Luther, Calvin, and Zwingli, placed a renewed emphasis on the doctrine of divine election, meaning that human faith, too, comes as a gift from God and is not possible apart from the divine grace of predestination. Luther also stressed the doctrine of *sola scriptura*, believing that scripture alone (rather than reason or church tradition) was the supreme rule of faith and life. What was not taught by scripture, with the aid of the Holy Spirit, was not authoritative. Scripture was given primacy over all human and ecclesiastical traditions and indeed over the church itself, a view that was summarized in the Reformation dictum *Ecclesia reformata semper reformanda* (The church reformed, always in need of reform).

The simultaneous existence of several strains of Protestantism guaranteed diversity within the movement. There was a degree of individual opinion even within each of the respective traditions, making it difficult to arrive at an authoritative position on many controverted issues of theology.[2] Yet despite these differences, all the branches that grew out of the Reformation agreed that the Catholic Church had over time created a theological and ecclesiastical superstructure that had obscured the original teachings of the early apostles as embodied in the New Testament. Basic to Protestantism was the doctrine of the priesthood of all believers, according to which all Christians can approach God personally and directly, without the mediation of a priest. The Catholic Church taught that salvation was mediated by the church through the administration of the sacraments. Moreover, in the Catholic tradition (in theory but not always in practice), only theologians and members of the priesthood could teach doctrine, while within Protestantism even laymen could write on theology. In Protestant countries natural philosophers penned treatises on the relationship of theology to science, physicians wrote on its relationship to medicine, and their ideas were widely read and respected. Yet when the layman Galileo (1564–1642) wrote on biblical interpretation in Catholic Italy, he was investigated by the Inquisition.

The Catholic Church summarized all doctrine in what came in the nineteenth century to be known as the Magisterium, which was the collection of the writings of the church fathers, papal encyclicals, and decrees of councils that constituted the official teaching of the church. There was no magisterium—no single authoritative body of teaching—within Protestantism. Protestantism was decentralized, taking a different form, that of the "territorial church," in each country. And Protestants were not subject to the Index of Prohibited Books (1516), by which the Catholic Church suppressed works that it regarded as heretical or dangerous to faith and morals. Nor did Protestants need fear the Inquisition, introduced at Rome in 1552 and active in some, but not all, Catholic countries in the sixteenth and seventeenth centuries, although enforcement was by no means uniform. In general, there was greater freedom of thought in Protestant than in Catholic countries.[3] Nevertheless, both were part of the same age, in which one risked one's life or liberty for actively promoting or even holding ideas that were perceived as heretical by their theological opponents.

Protestantism and Medicine

Given the Reformers' rejection of what they regarded as the superstitions of saints, relics, and pilgrimages, it is not surprising that Protestants rejected the miraculous healing practices that had been associated with them. The Reformers believed that miracles had ceased at the end of the age of the apostles (c. AD 100). Catholics, on the other hand, taught that God had given to the church the continuing gift of miracles, one of which was transubstantiation, the doctrine that in the Mass the bread and wine of the Eucharist are miraculously transformed into the body and blood of Christ.

Luther underplayed the role of miracles even in the New Testament. To him the preaching of the Word, conversion, and the transformation of lives under the impact of the gospel were more impressive than spectacular miracles. Luther held that, while the apostles had healed the sick by anointing them with oil, as in Mark 6:12–13, God no longer healed by oil and that the injunction in James 5:14–15 to heal by oil no longer applied to the church.

John Calvin (1509–1564) discussed the role of miracles in much greater detail. For him miracles were signs and seals that confirmed the truth of biblical revelation. But he argued that they had fulfilled their purpose in accrediting the ministry of the apostles and had therefore ceased.[4] This view became the common Protestant position, and it was widely held, though there were some exceptions, particularly among the founders of Protestant bodies that later grew up outside the churches of the Reformation. They include George Fox (1624–1691), who founded the Society of Friends (Quakers); Count Nikolaus von Zinzendorf (1700–1760), influential leader of the Moravians; and John Wesley, who founded the Methodist movement.[5]

But in times of stress and persecution some later Protestants also claimed to witness instances of supernatural healing. In *The Scots Worthies* (1774) John Howie described incidences of reported supernatural healing among the persecuted Scottish Covenanters in the seventeenth century. But Protestants tended to regard contemporary accounts of Catholic miracles as superstitious. Once the theology that undergirded the healing role of saints came under attack by Protestants, shrines and pilgrimage centers in Protestant regions of Europe fell into disrepute. The huge trade in fraudulent relics in the late Middle Ages and the wholesale hawking of indulgences to which Luther had objected had already prepared the way for a popular revulsion. In the reaction that followed the spread of Protestantism, piles of bones alleged to be those of saints were publicly burned. Healing shrines disappeared from northern Europe, though they continued in Catholic countries for centuries.

It has been much debated whether the spirit of early Protestantism had a formative influence on the scientific revolution of the sixteenth and seventeenth centuries.[6] It has been argued that the distrust of human traditions and ecclesiastical authority in matters of faith and religious practice extended to the sciences, where experimentation and the search for natural causes seemed to be a logical extension of the theological ideas of the Reformation. The Protestant Reformers certainly deeply respected medicine, as they did the sciences in general. Luther and Calvin accepted medicine (the correlative of a naturalistic understanding of disease) as a beneficial gift of God for the healing of disease and an expression of God's common grace to all humankind. "God created medicine and provided us with intelligence to guard and take care of the body so that we can live in good health," wrote Luther. But he also believed that when Satan was responsible for a disease, a "higher medicine, namely, faith and prayer" might be necessary.[7] Several anecdotes recorded in Luther's *Table Talk* refer to his praying for the healing of friends. A well-known instance is that of Friedrich Myconius, who in 1540 was on his deathbed when Luther prayed for his recovery. He recovered from his illness and survived Luther by two months, dying in 1546.

While Luther believed that God could and did heal in answer to prayer, Protestant theologians, like physicians, sought natural rather than supernatural causes of disease. When Ambroise Paré (1517?–1590), often called the father of modern surgery, uttered his famous dictum, "I dressed the patient, but God healed him" (Je le pansay et Dieu le guarit), he did not mean that God had acted miraculously in doing so. Elsewhere Paré stated that he confined his interest to "the natural causes of the plague" but left it to theologians to account for its ultimate cause. One early convert to Protestantism, Luther's associate Carlstadt, born Andreas Bodenstein (c. 1480–1541), broke with Luther over his own increasingly radical theological ideas, one of which was that Christians should look to God for healing through prayer rather than to medicine. Luther asked his burgomaster, who had been influenced by Carlstadt, whether he ate when he was hungry. When the burgomaster said that he did, Luther replied that he should also take medicine, which was as much God's gift as food and drink were. Protestant ideas of altruism and the spiritual utility of the secular professions, together with the value that Protestants placed on a learned ministry, combined to give the physician a respected status. Edinburgh, situated in strongly Presbyterian Scotland, produced what by the eighteenth century had become one of the finest medical faculties in Europe.[8]

Protestantism influenced the study of learned medicine in Germany, beginning in Luther's own university, the University of Wittenberg, where Philip Melanchthon (1497–1560), Luther's successor as the leader of the German Lutherans, was creating a new curriculum for Lutheran universities that reflected the spirit of both the Reformation and the Renaissance. Melanchthon regarded himself not merely as a religious reformer but as an educational one as well, and he extensively revised the undergraduate arts curriculum at Wittenberg along the lines of Renaissance humanism. His interest in natural theology led to his giving mathematics and astronomy a prominent place, because he believed that the heavens exhibited the beauty of God's creation.[9]

The mathematicians at Wittenberg were the earliest supporters of Copernicus in Europe, formulating the "Wittenberg interpretation," which relied on his more accurate tables for the movements of the heavenly bodies, while rejecting his heliocentric theory. Melanchthon regarded Copernicus as a reformer like himself. He lectured on natural philosophy and also introduced into the arts curriculum the new anatomy of another reformer, Vesalius (1514–1564), the founder of modern anatomy, together with the anatomical figures from his *De humani corporis fabrica* (*On the Fabric of the Human Body*, 1543), which Melanchthon had printed for his students in order to demonstrate God's handiwork in the human body. Vesalius had revolutionized the study of anatomy by rejecting the authority of Galen and by performing dissections himself.[10] Like other humanists, he attacked medical teachers' reliance on Latin translations of ancient Greek texts and Arab compendia in place of the personal examination (autopsy) of human anatomy that became common. Melanchthon thereby gave the new anatomy a broader influence among nonspecialists and provided the greater autonomy for their subject that anatomists desired in place of its previously inferior position as merely a surgical specialty. Although the curricular influence of the new "Wittenberg anatomy" spread to other northern European universities, by the seventeenth century Melanchthon's emphasis on anatomy had disappeared even in Wittenberg.

The widespread interest in the new anatomy fit well with a growing emphasis on the human body as a creation made in the image of God, the temple of the Holy Spirit, and the house of the immortal soul. Anatomy was also central to teleology, and knowledge of how the body worked had implications for understanding the soul. John Calvin admired the skill with which Galen had demonstrated the careful design of the body in his celebrated treatise *On the Usefulness of the Parts of the Human Body*. Catholics and Protestants agreed on anatomy's value as a pointer to the marvels of God's handiwork in nature. Natural history (the study of living forms of animals and plants), which focused largely on medicine, received an impetus from the enhanced religious sensitivity that emerged from the Protestant Reformation.[11]

Paracelsus and the Popularization of Medicine

The Protestant suspicion of ecclesiastical authority had its counterpart in medicine. Reform of university curricula and increased professional competence were in the air, and reformers in medicine abounded. Renaissance editions of the texts of Galen and other Greek and Latin medical writers encouraged learned physicians to challenge traditional medical knowledge. Learned physicians were a highly literate and cultured group. They were university-trained and had studied nature, which formed the basis of their understanding of the body; the name *physic* (medicine) derived from the Greek word for "nature," *phusis*.

One such medical reformer was Paracelsus, born Theophrastus von Hohenheim (1493–1541), a controversial medical innovator whom Catholics called, not intending it as a compliment, the "Luther of physicians" (*Luther medicorum*). Iconoclastic, quarrelsome, and egotistical, with an insatiable curiosity and wanderlust, he adopted the pen name Paracelsus ("Greater than Celsus," after the Roman writer on medicine). Paracelsus rejected the tradition of learned medicine and the idea that medicine could be acquired from books. Although a nominal Catholic, he came under the influence of two radical Protestant reformers, Sebastian Franck and Caspar Schwenckfeldt, who advocated social radicalism and an undogmatic Christianity outside the organized church. He penned an apocalyptic work, *Prophecy for the Next Twenty-four Years* (1536), which predicted a future marked by calamity that would end with the defeat of the Anti-Christ and the inauguration of the reign of God. He imbibed the empirical spirit of Protestantism and its rejection of traditional authority.[12]

After being appointed town physician and lecturer of medicine at Basel, Paracelsus caused a sensation by publicly burning Avicenna's *Canon*, which was widely used as a textbook in European faculties of medicine. Borrowing another page from Luther, who translated the Bible into the vernacular German, he announced that he would not lecture in Latin, preferring German instead. He was the first physician to refuse to lecture on Hippocrates and Galen, believing that medicine was given by God and not learned from books. A man of the Renaissance, he adopted the so-called occult (hidden) sciences, alchemy and astrology.[13]

The influence of Neoplatonism led Paracelsus to adopt an intuitive mystical approach that saw the world as full of spiritual and vital forces. He rejected the humoral pathology of Galen and sought instead the specific causes of disease, which he believed were the *archei*, spiritual entities that invaded the body and controlled bodily processes. Influenced by Protestant attacks on priestly authority, he condemned the medical practices of his time. He believed that God not only caused diseases but provided their cures as well. He also believed that God had placed drugs in minerals and that the poor could discover them without specialized knowledge and without the aid of expensive physicians. Anyone could read nature's book and practice medicine.

Paracelsus was influenced by the inductive approach of the Protestants even before it was encouraged in England by Bacon and his successors. Yet his quarrelsomeness and repudiation of learned medicine brought him into disfavor with the medical establishment. He was dismissed from Protestant Basel and could not find a teaching post anywhere else in Europe. Paracelsus's medical and alchemical works, published only after his death, came to have wide influence in high circles, especially among Protestants in northern Europe but also among Catholics in the medical faculty at Montpellier and at the French royal court. English Puritans adopted the Paracelsian system and sought a reform of medical education that would replace the writings of Aristotle and Galen with the iatro-chemistry of Paracelsus.

By the mid-seventeenth century a new scientific medicine was attempting to free itself from the tradition of Aristotle and Galen. The publication of *De motu cordis et sanguinis in animalibus* (*On the Motion of the Heart and Blood in Animals*), by William Harvey (1578–1657), in 1627 demonstrated irrefutably the circulation of the blood, "as it were, in a circle," the perfect motion that God had created. At the same time the medical profession attempted to create firmer boundaries to distinguish itself from other purveyors of health care on the basis of the new medicine.[14] There was no single scientific medicine, however, but rather a plethora of competing ideas, not all of them Paracelsian. Even Harvey refused to identify himself with the "new science."

As a reform movement Protestantism was fortunate to benefit from the Gutenberg Revolution. With the development of a moveable-type printing technology in the mid-fifteenth century, popular printing became widespread throughout Europe after 1500. It provided an efficient means for Protestants to disseminate their ideas, and Protestant theological ideas spread quickly throughout northern Europe. Less than two months after Luther posted his Ninety-five Theses in Wittenberg, they were being read by literate people throughout Germany in both Latin and German. Protestants were eager to propagate not only their theological doctrines but learning in general, including medicine.

The three centuries that followed the Reformation were an era of great medicalization, that is, the popularization of medicine among the masses. Initially this was done by medical elites, who held a low opinion of popular medical views. They thought that by spreading knowledge of medicine, they could free the laity from false notions of healing by superstition, white magic, and folk medicine.[15] Ignorance, which commonly led to illness, could be banished by the popularization of medically sound advice. Hence vade mecums that provided professional medical advice began to be widely published. Of course, there was plenty of popularization of unsound advice too. In England some books explicitly attacked the authority of Galen, extolling medical experience and the efficacy of native English drugs and arguing that the sick could treat themselves. Ecclesiasticus 38:4 was often cited in support of the common view that God had devised a remedy for every disease and that he had provided local remedies for local diseases. The related doctrine of signatures held that natural objects such as plants (e.g., liverwort) had distinguishing marks that indicated their efficacy for particular diseases, on the principle that like cures like. By contrast, Galenic medicine was allopathic, holding that disease was cured by its opposite.

But the medical elites who had authored books of popularized medicine were soon followed by more radical reformers, some of them inspired by Paracelsus, others by Protestants with an interest in challenging learned medicine, especially the older Galenic medicine. The most famous in England was the author of *Culpeper's Herbal*, Nicholas Culpeper (1616–1654), a Protestant who had fought on the side of Parliament in the English Civil War (1648–60). In 1652 he published *The English Physician*, an unauthorized translation of the pharmacopoeia of the College of Physicians, which was followed by his *Complete Herbal*. Culpeper attacked the learned medicine of physicians and relied, as he wrote, on "my two brothers, DR. REASON and DR. EXPERIENCE," to make medical knowledge available to all, particularly to the poor, who were unable to afford the expensive fees of doctors. In addition to using herbals (which often relieved symptoms or had a placebo effect), he incorporated astrology into medical therapy. Culpeper's *Herbal* remained a household guide to popular medicine for generations, becoming one of the most successful volumes of home remedies ever published.[16]

The Reform of Charity and Hospitals

As a result of the Protestant Reformation the treatment of the sick poor underwent considerable transformation in the sixteenth century toward secularization and, to some degree, medicalization.[17] In the Middle Ages, Christians had viewed the poor as being under the special care of God and as deserving objects of charity. Begging for alms was central to medieval charity, given the medieval understanding of evangelical poverty. The underlying theology was that poverty was a blessed estate that existed to remind those who had possessions of their own that they had a responsibility to assist those less fortunate. Their works of charity, moreover, provided a means of lessening their suffering in purgatory, an emphasis that was frequently primary in Catholic teaching. The rich engaged in good works by providing alms, while the poor earned their heavenly reward by begging and by praying for the soul of the almsgiver.

Luther and the Protestant Reformers attacked the mendicant religious orders, who sometimes begged for their living. They rejected the doctrine of voluntary poverty by challenging the theology on which it was based, the concept that good works could be meritorious for those performing them, and by arguing that it undercut genuine poverty, which communities should work to eliminate, as well as true charity, which should result from faith and love of one's neighbor rather than from the pursuit of salvation through works.[18] Protestants viewed begging as at best a temporary measure. While the sick poor had a justifiable claim on the assistance of the Christian community, they should seek to support themselves as soon as they were able to return to a normal life. Protestant countries limited or abolished begging for alms and replaced it with poor relief that was provided by municipal authorities in connection with the churches, in a joint effort in which overseers worked together with deacons. This became the pattern in the German cities, the United Provinces (Holland), England, Scotland (to a lesser extent), and the Scandinavian countries.

In the second half of the sixteenth century, authorities in Reformed and Lutheran countries and cities in northern Europe converted urban monasteries into secular lay institutions that were operated by municipalities for the poor and the sick. In England, Henry VIII had earlier confiscated the monasteries and closed their hospitals, which were placed under the control of secular boards. Catholic religious orders were laicized, while nuns were released from their vows and forbidden to distribute alms. In Calvin's Geneva, the city consolidated the hospitals, together with other charitable institutions, to form the General Hospital, which was operated as a municipal institution. Converting monasteries into municipally operated hospitals and merging several smaller hospitals into larger ones were the most common Protestant approaches to hospital maintenance. The underlying basis for doing so, however, was not to remove religious motivation from charity but to create a Christian commonwealth that took upon itself the obligation to provide medical care for the destitute, with the intent of creating productive citizens of society.

An ideological basis for the reforms was provided by several Protestant theologians and by Christian humanists as well. Both advocated programmatic poor relief to those who were morally upright residential members of the community (as opposed to being vagrants). Prominent among these theologians was Andreas Hyperius (1511–1564), a professor of theology at Marburg and a noted humanist, whose *De publica in pauperes beneficentia* (*Public Beneficence among the Poor*, 1570) was translated into English and encouraged the role of medical care in poor relief, which took on a major role in Protestant reforms. In England, as in Protestant cities on the Continent, poor relief and health care were centralized in common institutions, which included both hospitals, which were often situated in former monasteries, and workhouses, in which, unfortunately, "workers" too often lived in unsanitary and abusive conditions.

The rationale was theological and had been provided initially by the Protestant Reformers. Luther's views were popularized in his early treatise *Letter to the Christian Nobility of the German Nation* (1520). Ulrich Zwingli (1484–1531), the leading Protestant Reformer in Zurich, called the involuntary poor "living images of God" and urged poor relief so that "Christ should lie no more abroad in the streets." The duty to help the sick and the poor was a staple of Protestant sermons and pamphlets by which pastors encouraged their congregations to give liberally to assist those in need. But it constituted only one aspect of the Reformers' goal of transforming both church and society.

Protestant reforms of the mode of baptizing infants and the regulation of midwifery, as demonstrated by the work of Johannes Bugenhagen (1485–1558), a close friend and collaborator of Luther's who designed an extensive program of poor relief, had broader implications for health.[19] Of course, the new institutions and regulations provided a good deal of social control, as Foucault has emphasized. But as Ole Grell and other leading social historians of medicine have noted, the historical sources leave little doubt that care was the primary motivation. Protestants' concern supported the claim of the Reformers to bring about nothing less than a wholesale reconstitution of the Christian community on Christian principles.[20]

Economic and social factors brought about a transformation in traditional attitudes toward the poor. A rapid population increase in the sixteenth century led to crowded cities, while repeated crop failures and resultant famine in rural areas led to masses of starving peasants leaving the countryside for cities. Wages fell and food prices rose, with a resulting increase in the number of poor vagabonds. Regular outbreaks of the plague through the early modern era were another major contributing factor to the socioeconomic crisis. Municipal authorities began to organize poor relief by channeling monies from scattered charitable institutions into a common fund modeled on Luther's Common Chest or by introducing poor rates (taxes for the charitable support of the poor), as was done in England and Holland. In municipalities where religious populations were mixed, Catholics and Protestants often cooperated to create municipal services to carry out this program.

Basic to the change in hospital care were the substitution of secular for religious support of charity and an administrative desire to manage the numerous poor. Holy Spirit hospitals, founded in late medieval times to care for both the poor and the sick, survived the Reformation. In southern Germany in the sixteenth century several such hospitals were founded in both Protestant and Catholic towns as charitable multipurpose institutions that served religious, social, and political functions. They became centers for care of the sick poor, distributing food to prevent pestilence and providing shelter not only for those who were sick or in need but for those who were healthy as well. They also admitted for short stays those who had suffered trauma. Over time they became increasingly diversified in treatment and types of patients.[21]

Charitable institutions not infrequently found themselves short of funds after the Reformation, and it has been argued that the motivation for Protestant charity might have been less effective than the motivation offered by Catholic theology. For a half-century after the Reformation, Protestant monarchs considered public charity to be an aspect of their religious duties. By the late 1580s, however, crown grants proved to be inadequate and were replaced by private endowments. As municipal institutions, hospitals increasingly had to depend for their financial resources on private charity, though churches also provided support.

No part of continental Europe was better known for its welfare institutions than the Netherlands, where the Reformed churches worked closely with municipal authorities. But the fact that the English were able to introduce a poor rate, while Continental countries failed to do so, is one that Grell attributes to a "long Reformation [that] carried with it a special dynamic which repeatedly served to inspire new generations of Protestants." After several earlier but unsuccessful attempts, the English Poor Law, championed by leading Puritans in Parliament, was established in 1601. It tied poor relief and medical care to parish life and placed both under the care of parish clergy and officers. It required that workhouses be established in major cities to regulate behavior by discouraging idleness among healthy and able-bodied beggars and ensuring that vagrants and vagabonds, who were thought to be carriers of epidemic diseases, would be confined. Outdoor (extra-institutional) relief of the poor was maintained by a poor rate that would be levied on each house in the parish and collected jointly by municipal and church authorities. The authorities did not always distribute charity gratis within the parish, since whenever possible they asked the able-bodied poor to assist in the care of the sick as part of their duty to society, a system that worked reasonably well. The goal was cure rather than long-term care so that the sick could return to a productive life. Care was local and therefore varied widely from place to place.[22]

Hospital care changed in Catholic countries as well. In Italy, famous hospitals that had once served as hospices for travelers and the healthy poor had come, by the early sixteenth century, to limit their care to the sick poor. But the treatment varied. The most famous hospital in Europe, Santa Maria Nuova in Florence, still enjoyed its superior reputation at the end of the century. Even with the secularization of hospitals during the Renaissance, the care of the soul retained its primary importance, with the theme of Christus medicus central to the healing of both soul and body. This may be illustrated by the manner in which the hospital's statutes describe the care given to a dying patient:

> When a patient is close to death, we place before him an image of Christ on the cross, and a nurse watches over him, never leaving his side and reading him the Creed, the Lord's Passion, and other holy texts. When he is dead, the head nurse comes with assistants; they take the dead man from the bed, clothe him in linen, and place him on a bier in the middle of the ward, where the chapel is, with a consecrated candle at his head and a lamp at his feet. At the appointed time a bell rings, and the priest comes with a cross. Two lay brothers light torches and the others take the body and bear it to the church, where the funeral service is sung.[23]

In the sixteenth century the new ideas advocated by Catholic reformers, such as Ignatius Loyola (1491 or 1495–1556), gained increasing acceptance, as their ideas came to be recognized as conforming to scripture and the church's historic teachings. In 1531 Charles V issued an ordinance that encouraged reforms in the Netherlands. In France, monarchs placed hospitals under secular directors, as Louis XII did the Hôtel-Dieu, in Paris, in 1505 and as Charles IX did in the case of village hospitals later in the century. In spite of this, Catholic sisters continued to carry out nursing duties, since most laypeople were unwilling to perform the menial tasks hospitals required.

The reorganization of hospitals not only marked a transition from medieval charity to a civic and secular social policy but also produced a change in the way society viewed the poor. Since the first Christian charitable organization, in the fourth century, the poor had been viewed as especially set apart by God and deserving of care. Now they became divided into the deserving and the undeserving poor, a distinction first found in legislation passed in Denmark in 1522. The undeserving poor were perceived as disease-ridden vagabonds and beggars who refused to work and who introduced infection into the city, thereby posing a threat to the social order. They were routinely sent back to their cities of birth. But society also recognized the deserving poor as a separate category made up of children, widows, and the aged who were thought to have suffered misfortune and therefore deserved public assistance. Where institutional resources permitted, those thought to deserve public assistance were placed in hospitals and workhouses and provided with medical care; where resources were lacking or facilities were overcrowded, they were given assistance on the streets. This new way of viewing the poor is still widely prevalent in Western society.[24]

In the seventeenth century, the Counter Reformation, the reform movement in the Catholic Church that followed the Protestant Reformation, produced a surge of religious charity, much of it centered on Vincent de Paul (c. 1580–1660), who encouraged many relief efforts among the sick and the poor. One by-product of the new interest was a profusion of self-help manuals. *The Charitable Remedies*, by Madame Fouquet, which was the best-known of them, enjoyed such popularity that it continued to be reprinted and used well into the nineteenth century.[25]

The most notable feature of the resurgence of Catholic medical charity, however, was the seventeenth-century reform of the French system of hospitals and related charitable institutions. The Catholic Company of the Holy Sacrament, which began in the 1620s, succeeded in constructing more than one hundred *hôpitaux-généraux* (general hospitals) in France in the second half of the seventeenth century. Altogether they housed more than one hundred thousand of the sick, the aged, and those who could not help themselves. In 1633 the most famous of all Catholic nursing orders, the Sisters of Charity, was founded by Vincent de Paul and Louise de Marillac. The order was the first congregation of women entirely devoted to caring for the sick and the poor. (Nuns had previously been cloistered and kept from working outside the walls of the convent.) The Sisters of Charity were drawn from all classes, the wealthy as well as the poor, and trained to serve as practical nurses. Real medical care in hospitals was still to come, but the sisters provided palliative care in the slums of Paris. Dressed in their distinctive religious habit with the signature winged coif that came to emblemize French medical charity, they brought assistance to the poor outside the cloister. By 1789 the Sisters of Charity had founded 426 houses throughout France. Many religious orders established after the death of Vincent de Paul followed the Vincentian model.[26]

Women in Medicine

In Tudor and Stuart England, much of the medical treatment was furnished by unlicensed or irregular practitioners who in many cases were women. University-trained physicians tended to congregate in large cities. Since a university education was not open to women, they could not be called physicians. They commonly served as midwives and were often employed by local governments, usually in offering ancillary medical services to the poor. For example, during the 1570s the city of Norwich employed women to provide about one-third of all medical treatment for the poor.

Women occasionally were found in irregular medical practice at a high level, especially in Paracelsian medicine, which members of the gentry administered as unlicensed practitioners. This traditional role among upper-class woman continued over several centuries. Women might acquire some knowledge of medicine (Galenic, Paracelsian, or astrological, but especially folkloric) in order to deal with needs within their family as well as among the tenants on their estates. They often kept journals, in which they passed down recipes to their daughters and nieces. Some of them helped in childbirth, dressed wounds, and made their own medications. Others kept herb gardens and practiced alchemy.

One such woman was Lady Grace Mildmay (1552–1620), whose autobiography, diary, and extensive personal and medical papers have allowed Linda Pollock to reconstruct in detail her life as a sixteenth-century English gentlewoman practicing nonprofessional medicine. Lady Mildmay was a deeply devout Anglican of Puritan sympathies who spent much time each day reading the Bible and works of devotion. She kept a spiritual diary and devoted part of each day to personal meditation. In addition, as she writes, "every day I spent some time in the herbal and books of physic, and in ministering to one or other by the directions of the best physicians of my acquaintance."[27]

Lady Mildmay devoted a good deal of her time to giving medical attention to all in her village who needed her help. She made herbal remedies on a fairly large scale from both chemicals and minerals, assembling altogether a collection of 270 medications. She did a good deal of medical reading, and she mentions some authors by name in connection with her remedies, such as Avicenna's syrup, which she found effective for melancholy. She had several popular books of medicine and collections of regimens. Fascinated by the new iatrochemistry, she corresponded with other alchemical practitioners. But although she was herself an alchemist, her practice was more dependent on Galenic than on Paracelsian methods. She used regimens that treated the whole body and focused on alleviating symptoms. Each regimen was suited to her patient's age, sex, and physical strength. Unlike some women practitioners, she did not perform surgery or remove cataracts, but she did treat illnesses such as frenzy and madness by medical means, employing diet, purges, vomiting, and bloodletting. She had what was in effect an apothecary's shop and a small medical library, as well as more than two thousand loose medical papers.

Although not a medically trained or learned practitioner, Lady Mildmay administered therapy that was not different in kind from that offered by trained physicians. Indeed, recent scholarship has stressed the overlap that existed between licensed and unlicensed practitioners. For that reason, to call her an "amateur" misrepresents both her own autodidactic skills and those of trained professionals. Of course, only upper-class and educated women had the time and resources to engage in medicine in the way that Lady Milmay did. But there were poor women who practiced medicine on a much lower level in villages and rural areas, though without the advantages of access to medical treatises and the ingredients with which to mix recipes.

The increasing insistence that physicians be licensed led to the medical profession's gradual exclusion of irregular practitioners. Women were increasingly forbidden to serve as apprentices. If they continued to practice medicine, they could not take fees. Hence they came to be associated with charlatans, and their practice was limited to women and children. Women employed in hospitals and orphanages were often little more than domestics, a position that required no special training. They worked in institutions that housed recipients of charity, such as the poor, the handicapped, and foundling children. Conditions and wages were poor, and the work was usually an extension of women's work in the home.

Health, Sickness, and Suffering

In general, Protestants, like most Christians, regarded the body as a relative, not an absolute, good. Health was not a virtue (as it was for the Greeks), but a blessing bestowed by God. Both Martin Luther and John Calvin echoed a widely held Christian view in arguing that good health, like every other human condition, could be used either for God's glory or for selfish purposes. But they also introduced what were to become distinctively Protestant convictions. On the one hand, the Reformers explicitly rejected monastic practices that sought to mortify the body as a meritorious work. At the same time, Protestants urged care for the body, since it was both God's workmanship and the temple of the Holy Spirit, a perspective that encouraged a milder strain of asceticism that found its expression in abstinence and moderation. This asceticism varied from tradition to tradition, receiving its greatest emphasis in Pietism and Methodism, as well as in the Holiness movements that grew out of Methodism.[28] Thus the early Methodists, under the influence of Francis Asbury (1745–1816), discouraged (as did the Quakers) the use of substances like tobacco and alcohol as incompatible with biblical standards of holiness.

Basic to Protestant understandings of health-related matters was the belief, which Protestants shared with most orthodox Christians, that sickness and suffering were a permanent element of the human condition.[29] Christians lived in a fallen world that was corrupted by the effects of original sin, of which disease and bodily suffering were a part. No Protestant Reformer or orthodox theologian within the Protestant tradition could anticipate a future in this life in which disease would be fully eliminated. In the present world, sin was always present, and with it the curse of physical suffering. Only in the final resurrection would Christians be given new, heavenly bodies and would death, the final enemy, be conquered. In the meantime, medicine offered alleviation of suffering, as well as progress in overcoming it. But if disease and pain were evils, Protestants believed that they were used by God incidentally to produce beneficial spiritual effects—to purify from sin, to soften hearts, to sensitize to spiritual concerns, to create sympathy for others who experienced suffering, and (especially central to Luther's thought) to increase trust of and dependence on God and to discourage self-sufficiency.

Calvinists in particular took a providential view of life that found a place in God's plan for illness and affliction. Believing firmly in God's sovereignty over human affairs, they looked for the hand of God in the everyday occurrences of their lives. The potential benefits of affliction led those striving to be godly to develop a keen eye for suffering in themselves and others. Thus Cotton Mather's (1663–1728) *Magnalia Christi Americana* (*The Great Works of Christ in America,* 1702) devotes a major section to biographies of New England's founders, many of which detail suffering as contributing to the founders' Christian character.

But in spite of much popular opinion to the contrary, Protestant theologians did not consider most disease and physical suffering to be God's retributive punishment for personal sin. Since Christ had already borne the punishment for sin by his death on the cross, disease did not have to be a sign of God's displeasure toward the sufferer but could be God's discipline of his disobedient child. The danger existed, however, that in the midst of one's suffering one might become so focused on one's pain as to neglect spiritual concerns. This was a concern of Cotton Mather's in both his *Angel of Bethesda* (the first medical book written in America, though it was not published until the twentieth century) and his personal diary.[30]

Vocation and Conscience

Protestantism approached the Christian life somewhat differently than did traditional Catholicism. In place of the monastic ideal of an ascetic or reclusive life, it encouraged Christians to combine attention to personal holiness with active service in the world. Central to the Reformers' view of the spiritual life was the idea of vocation. Medieval Catholic theologians had divided the world into spiritual and temporal estates, with those who desired to serve God fully seeking a vocation as a priest or, within the contemplative life, as a monk or nun, while secular professions (the active life) were regarded as distinctly second best. Luther and Calvin abolished for Protestants the medieval distinction between sacred and secular callings, seeing both as possibilities for all Christians. All professions had the potential to be spiritually fulfilling. A physician who sought to glorify God through medicine could play as important a role in society as a minister. Hence Protestantism encouraged the participation of Christians in every aspect of society, with the confidence that they could provide a redemptive force in a sinful world. Their confidence was rooted, not in aspirations of transforming the world by human effort, but in a firm belief that ordinary human activity, no matter how humble, could serve as an outworking of redeeming grace. In medicine, Protestant physicians and philosophers as well as theologians—laymen as well as clergy—influenced the formulation of medical ethics.[31]

Protestantism rejected the formulation of a detailed system of ethics and rolled ethics back into systematic theology. Protestant medical ethics arose more directly from religious considerations of health and disease, as well as from biblical themes like providence, justification, law and grace, covenant, and the place of suffering in Christian experience. Hence Protestantism produced no tradition of casuistry such as that found in the Catholic Church.[32] Some early Anglicans and Puritans, however, penned manuals on "cases of conscience," of which Richard Baxter's (1615–1691) *Christian Directory* is a representative example. In addressing the duties of physicians (pt. 4, ch. 5), Baxter, a Puritan minister who also practiced medicine, urged physicians to make "the honouring and pleasing [of] God, and the public good, and the saving of men's lives" their intention rather than their own honor or profit. He advised them to help the poor, to seek the counsel of abler physicians in difficult cases, to rely on God for direction and success, to avoid atheism (a danger to which physicians were widely believed to be prone), and to use opportunities to speak to their patients, especially dying patients, of their souls.[33]

The development of a tradition of Protestant casuistry was hindered, however, by elements inherent in the nature of Protestantism. Beginning with Luther, many Protestants retained a strong antipathy toward anything that resembled the constraints of legalism, while they largely, though not entirely, ignored the long tradition of natural law that had played such an important role in Catholic moral theology. Their rejection of private confession and penance further weakened the development of casuistic ethics. Perhaps their negative reaction to the highly developed tradition of casuistry within Catholicism was enough to weaken the attempt to create a similar tradition among Protestants. Instead, Protestants stressed commandment and conscience, or norm and context—the application of general biblical principles, such as those of the Decalogue, to particular situations—as the twin pillars on which ethics should be based.

The individual alone before God was a basic Protestant theme. The cultivation of the private conscience, which sought to apply the text of scripture to concrete ethical situations, became a characteristic emphasis. This approach was ideally suited to the Baconian tradition of English (and later American) Protestantism. Francis Bacon (1561–1626) believed that induction was the most fruitful method of acquiring scientific knowledge. Eschewing the deductive method and all-embracing explanatory systems, he urged the patient building of knowledge on secure empirical foundations. The empirical and inductive premises of the Baconian tradition influenced later British thinkers and institutions, especially Robert Boyle (1627–1691) and the Royal Society, which was founded in 1660. In the eighteenth century the Scottish philosophy of common sense, which was rooted in Baconianism as well as in natural-law theory, found ready acceptance among Anglo-Saxon Protestants, who applied the inductive method both to the interpretation of scripture and to the construction of theological and ethical systems on the basis of biblical texts, while avoiding excessive speculation.[34]

Professional Medical Ethics

While pre-nineteenth-century medical literature contains little discussion of what we should term *medical ethics*, its allusion to the ideals of the profession of medicine is tinged with religious and moral values. The physician was expected to be an educated gentleman and to observe the precepts of Christian behavior. Character was essential in allowing him to fulfill the professional responsibilities that accompanied a high calling. A physician enjoyed opportunities to give counsel in spiritual matters and to admonish patients of the need for repentance or moral improvement. The analogy between healing bodies and healing souls was one that went back to the Greeks. Society expected Christian doctors to provide a form of spiritual service. Medicine was a humane art that was especially open to opportunities for beneficence on the part of those who viewed it as a calling in the service of God. While this ideal was by no means limited to Protestants, the personal response of the physician was of primary importance, given the Protestant aversion to casuistry in moral theology and the lack of canon law to give guidance. For generations of Protestant physicians, a sense of Christian duty took the place of an external code of ethics.[35]

From the sixteenth through the eighteenth century, many Protestant clergymen practiced medicine on the side. In the early seventeenth century Lutheran pastors in Denmark often studied basic medicine because they were expected to minister in rural areas, where physicians would be rare. According to Andrew Wear, "Protestant reformers in England during the Civil War period of the 1640s hoped to reorganize medical provision and to create a nationwide health service centered around clergymen who would act as physicians, their learning and sense of charity making them, in the eyes of the reformers, eminently qualified for such a role." Cleric-physicians flourished especially in rural parishes and small towns, where trained physicians were rare and clergymen had the leisure and learning to read medical books. In many towns ministers made up the only university-educated class, and they enjoyed great respect for their ability to offer medical healing. Although some undertook medical practice to supplement their income, most did so for humanitarian reasons or to increase their respect in the community, and many accepted no fees for their services. One seventeenth-century Anglican minister, Richard Napier, rector of the parish of the small town of Great Linford, Buckinghamshire, spent most of his time practicing medicine, while his curate took over preaching. There were no physicians in the town, and in his career of forty-one years Napier treated some sixty thousand patients.[36]

Puritan and Separatist ministers often showed a special interest in medicine. In colonial New England, ministers who were engaged in medical practice were so common in towns and villages outside Boston that Cotton Mather, of Boston, himself a minister who practiced medicine, referred to the care of soul and body as the "angelical conjunction." "O though *Afflicted*," wrote Mather, "and under Distemper, Go to *Physicians* in *Obedience* to God, who has commanded the *Use of Means*. But place thy *Dependence* on God alone to Direct and Prosper them. And know, that they are *Physicians of no* Value, if He do not so. . . . *Tis from God, and not from the Physician, that my Cure is to be looked for*."[37]

Mather became the center of controversy when, during an epidemic of smallpox in 1721, he supported the physician Zabdiel Boylston, who inoculated against the disease. Together with the local press, conservative physicians such as Dr. William Douglass, an Edinburgh graduate, opposed the controversial practice as medically unsafe and Mather's advocacy as clerical interference in medicine. Five other prominent members of the clergy supported Mather. Other pioneering pastors in colonial America assumed medical treatment of Indians and European settlers where there were no doctors.

John Wesley (1703–1791) took a course in medicine before he departed for America in 1735 so that as a minister he could be of help to those who had no regular physician. After two years of ministering in Georgia, he returned to England. In 1746, after observing the lack of medical care among his parishioners, he opened a dispensary that employed an apothecary and a surgeon. In the next year he published a lay medical guide, *Primitive Physick*, in the tradition of every man his own physician, which sold for one shilling and enjoyed wide circulation. Wesley popularized the ideas of Dr. George Cheyne, particularly regarding the influence of diet on health, which became a part of Wesley's "method" for holy living, a component of the Methodist movement. Wesley believed that his approach constituted a return to a "primitive," or simple, empirical approach to medicine that was unencumbered by theory. The book, which recommended "only safe and cheap and easy" remedies for some three hundred diseases, had undergone twenty-three editions by the time of Wesley's death in 1791, and it was still being reprinted in the 1970s.[38]

Clergymen frequently took the initiative in matters of public health. In 1822 the Catholic archbishop of Paris urged the priests of his dioceses to assist local authorities in vaccination efforts against smallpox. When James Young Simpson (1811–1870) introduced chloroform as an anesthetic in Edinburgh in 1847, religious criticism was virtually nonexistent. It was supported by many clergymen, including the distinguished Scottish theologian Thomas Chalmers. The chief opposition came from physicians, who adduced medical, ethical, and safety objections.[39]

Protestant Moral Theology

There are few examples in early Protestantism of disputed questions that anticipated modern medical-ethical concerns, and they fall properly under the rubric of moral theology. One was the matter of suicide. Augustine's (354–430) view that suicide was a violation of the sixth commandment, forbidding murder, and a sin that precluded repentance (*City of God* 1.17–27) was almost universally accepted by Catholic moral theologians in early modern Europe. While most Protestants also accepted the Augustinian formulation, some contended that suicides suffering from melancholy or insanity might ultimately experience God's forgiveness. John Sym (1581?–1637), in *Lifes Preservative Against Self-Killing* (1637), and John Donne (1572–1631), in *Biathanatos* (written in 1607 or 1608 for private circulation), argued for the latter position. Donne asserted that suicide was not the "irremissible" sin that Christian teaching made it out to be, and his work provoked much debate. His position was challenged by several authors, but others (chiefly Anglicans and Puritans) maintained that God might indeed forgive suicide in exceptional cases and that one should not judge the state of the heart.[40]

The question was never resolved among Protestants of that era, but the debate that followed assumed what was to become a familiar Protestant pattern. Certain moral questions did not permit easy solution, because the biblical evidence was not clear. In such cases Protestants drew inferences either from biblical principles or from passing references in scripture. But Protestants were willing to remain silent where scripture did. This meant that they were more inclined than Catholics to admit exceptions and to entrust doubtful cases to the judgment and mercy of God. The difference is nicely illustrated by a discussion that took place in 1600 between the Anglican George Abbot, future archbishop of Canterbury, and a Catholic Jesuit, John Gerard, regarding whether suicide was an unforgivable sin. Gerard described the discussion as follows:

> "But," said the doctor, "we don't know whether this was such a sin."
> "Pardon me," I said, "it is not a case here of our judgement. It is a question

of God's judgement; He forbids us under pain of hell to kill anyone, and particularly ourselves, for charity begins at home."

The good doctor was caught. He said nothing more on the point.[41]

This approach, the almost inevitable outcome of the Protestant method of dealing with controverted issues in moral theology, remains a common one to this day.

Tridentine Catholicism

The Catholic Church, after initial confusion and disarray, reacted vigorously to the Protestant Reformation. It addressed the abuses in the church, which Catholic reformers themselves admitted were many, and also gave an official formulation of many traditional Catholic understandings pertaining to theological matters. Both were undertaken by the Council of Trent, which met intermittently from 1545 to 1563. The doctrinal formulations of Trent determined the theological and moral stance of the Catholic Church for the next four hundred years, until the Second Vatican Council (1962–65).

At the center of contrasting theologies was the church's understanding of sin. "Trent . . . differed from the Protestant reformers in seeing original sin as debilitating rather than as radically destructive. It differed from them also in relating grace to human merit and striving. The council proclaimed the essential freedom of the human will."[42] These distinctions were crucial in defining faith and practice within the Tridentine (post-Trent) Catholic tradition. The gospel was to be spread in ways that appealed to the senses, such as through the sacraments, images, architecture, preaching, and catechizing. Trent affirmed the contribution of good works to personal salvation, as well as the objective efficacy of the seven sacraments, which convey grace *ex opere operato*, that is, by the simple act of being administered. The Eucharistic sacrifice, in which the priest miraculously transformed the wafer and wine on the altar into the body and blood of Christ, remained central to Catholic liturgy and piety and the most important focus in the weekly cycle of Catholic Christians.

This admixture of spirit and matter, seen most notably in God's acting through the sacraments, was important in the Catholic conception of the healing of disease and the care of the sick. It tied healing to ritual and permitted the continued use of what Protestants termed "superstitious" practices, such as reliance on relics, pilgrimages, and the intercession of saints (including living saints), to flourish, though the church struggled to regulate them. *Tolerari potest*, "Let it be allowed," was a common response by the clergy to popular healing practices, but the line between acceptable and unacceptable was a fine one, and the church reserved to itself the right to determine it.

The Protestant Reformation and the attacks of satirists like Erasmus had lessened the flow of pilgrims to the great healing centers in Protestant countries, but alternative forms of pilgrimage, such as imaginary pilgrimages in one's own home, became popular. The widespread appeal of relics and miracles continued long after the Reformation, however. Santiago became more prosperous in the seventeenth century than it had been in the Middle Ages, and the cult of saints continued to enjoy popularity in Catholic Europe well into the eighteenth century, testifying to the survival of medieval piety when the Reformation might have been expected to strike it a fatal blow. Healing by means of relics remained a staple of Catholic folk piety even when its claims of alleged miracles sometimes embarrassed educated Catholics. These claims often involved popular religious practices that dated back to pre-Christian times. In some cases they represented a syncretistic element of animism or paganism, and they could be found in every country in which Catholicism flourished. While they represented unofficial devotions, popular enthusiasm, or folk or magical practices, because they were tolerated by local priests or the hierarchy they became part of the Catholic world. But the church had an elaborate procedure for determining genuine miracles of healing by candidates for canonization. Such miracles reflected that aspect of Catholicism that emphasized sacramental action through ritual ceremonies in every aspect of life.[43]

In Tridentine Catholicism the seminary-trained parish priest spent most of his time administering the sacraments, preaching, and hearing confessions. In some parishes he also practiced medicine, carrying on the tradition of clerical medicine (*medicina clericalis*) that dated from the Middle Ages. Although medieval prohibitions against clerics' practicing medicine theoretically remained in force, they were relaxed in the seventeenth century, especially among missionaries, who regarded medicine as a means of facilitating conversion. In the eighteenth century, clerical medicine underwent a revival under the encouragement of Continental secular governments that hoped to use the clergy to administer medical assistance in their parishes. A manual even appeared to help the parish priest treat a variety of conditions, including childbirth. As confessor he could not have any illusions about the deeply rooted influence of original sin on those to whom he ministered. But he hoped that the penitential system, the backbone of Catholic moral theology and the church's means of creating among them a spirit of contrition, would eventually lead to an abandoning of sinful habits.[44]

Against the Protestant doctrine of *sola fide*, Trent reiterated the doctrine that in addition to faith, good works were necessary to salvation. The theology of merit (one's hope to be rewarded by God for one's good works) from a certain point developed into an important motivator of the church's charitable activities, and it continued to inspire them in the seventeenth century. In France the government employed rural priests to assist in distributing medicines that the central government had sent to their parishes. The clergy also assisted the government during times of epidemic. But the growing professionalism of doctors ultimately brought about the end of clerical medicine in Europe, while in America by the end of the nineteenth century every state had enacted legislation that prevented clergy who had no medical training from practicing medicine. The legislation was motivated by the desire of physicians to establish a monopoly by excluding irregular practitioners.[45]

The Enlightenment

Historians often speak of the "long" eighteenth century, which by extension dates from 1648 (the end of the Thirty Years' War) to 1815 (the defeat of Napoleon).[46] The eighteenth-century Enlightenment began in France and spread throughout the Continent, as well as to England, Scotland, and America. A general definition that covers all those who held Enlightenment assumptions is impossible. Enlightenment thinking differed in degree from country to country and varied according to one's religious predilections, from rationalistic theism to deism to atheism. The spirit of enlightenment was the result of the scientific and intellectual developments of the previous century. It popularized the ideas of Isaac Newton, John Locke, Francis Bacon, and René Descartes. It was an age that was critical of religion and confident in the ability of human reason and science to provide answers to matters that previously had been explained by religion.

During the eighteenth century, reason replaced belief in divine revelation among many but by no means all European intellectuals. Rather than viewing faith and reason as complementary, elites began to speak of reason as opposed to faith. Rationalism, the belief that human reason alone was capable of answering scientific and philosophical questions and resolving problems, became widely accepted. Mechanistic ideas had been adopted in some form by most philosophers by the end of the seventeenth century and greatly influenced the scientific enterprise. The Baconian model gave researchers confidence that science was capable of producing infinite technological progress.

The Enlightenment was characterized by a widespread desire for rational planning of society and the economy and for secular initiatives that were undertaken by the state. Scientific societies, such as the Royal Society in London, the Académie royale des sciences in Paris, and the Leopoldina in Vienna, as well as journals, such as the *Philosophical Transactions of the Royal Society*, enjoyed enormous prestige, and they supported progressive ideas in every area. On the other hand, religious belief continued and even grew in many places in Europe, and its decline, where it occurred, has generally been overestimated. In medicine in particular, religious ideas continued to be influential. It is a mistake to consider the Enlightenment a period marked by intellectual and antireligious homogeneity.

Enlightenment Medicine

Since the Vincentian reforms of charity and the organization of the Sisters of Charity, Catholic nursing orders, many of them Augustinian, had formed the nursing staff of French hospitals. After the French Revolution the new government secularized hospitals and disbanded religious orders, though they found it difficult to carry on adequate nursing without the Catholic sisters, who viewed their service as compassionate care of the needy. Their views conflicted with the Enlightenment role of the hospital as an institution for bringing about medical progress. The Hôtel-Dieu, in Paris, had once housed as many as three thousand patients at a time, but concern for their care gave way to the advance of scientific medicine, which created one of the most famous schools of medicine in the world. The role of the hospital changed as well, becoming one of contributing to the mercantilist policies of European governments in restoring the health of the working population. In mercantilist theory, the population of a nation was its most valuable resource, furnishing a steady supply of labor for national industry and military service.[47]

The emphasis on the sufficiency of human reason and an optimistic belief in human progress furnished an impetus for the pursuit of advancement in medicine, particularly in northern Europe, where the spirit of the Enlightenment encouraged empiricism and rationalism. The optimism of Enlightenment thinkers led to the belief that disease could be controlled or prevented by rational application of diet, medicine, and behavior. No longer regarded as a permanent element of the human condition, disease was viewed instead as a condition to be eliminated through progress in medicine. Medical professionals saw their role expanded considerably in order to assist governmental and professional bodies in creating a comprehensive and systematic program of medical health.

Mechanistic ideas influenced medical investigators to pursue a variety of theoretical approaches in which physicians took the lead. Many distinguished Enlightenment figures were physicians; their empirical approach to medicine encouraged them to expand the boundaries of knowledge, which they often did, not merely in medicine but in a variety of areas. Physicians were expected, by the standards of the time, to dedicate themselves to the improvement of mankind. In their medical research, naturalistic models of disease replaced a religious outlook. While they focused their research on understanding the human body, they frequently went beyond that focus in attempting to construct a science of man, always pursuing an empirical rather than a philosophical (deductive) approach, and always expecting progress to be made. Peter Gay suggests that "for observant men in the eighteenth century, philosophes as well as others, the most tangible cause for confidence [in human progress] lay in medicine."[48]

The Enlightenment encouraged new emphases that considerably expanded tendencies that already existed. One was on the expansion of health care by the state, which first developed as a conscious program in the eighteenth century. This involved attention to public-health measures and improving the environment in which people lived by, for example, draining swamps and ensuring clean drinking water. Governments became involved in informing their subjects, particularly peasants, about issues of health and hygiene in a variety of genres, including the question-and-answer format commonly used for religious catechisms, such as Bernard Faust's, written for schools in the German state of Hesse. Emphasis was also placed on the individual's responsibility for his or her own health, and self-help was encouraged. A plethora of manuals offered advice for maintaining one's health, which had long been a characteristic feature of European society but which received new emphasis in the Enlightenment.

Despite widespread anticlericalism, priests were regarded as a first line of defense against disease in poor and rural parishes in France. Samuel Auguste Tissot, in a manual written to help priests provide basic medical care for their parishioners, gave health-related advice and warned against debilitating moral habits, such as drink and masturbation. During the Enlightenment there were a number of efforts to revive clerical medicine as a means of extending medical care to the poor, one of the few priestly duties that rationalists thought beneficial. Johann Peter Frank, of the University of Vienna, who created the most efficient health-care system in Europe, was also the most energetic in developing plans to use priests as clerical physicians. In Sweden, the celebrated botanist Carl von Linné (Carolus Linnaeus) proposed, without success, that every theology student be given a short course on medicine. In Russia, Czar Alexander I decreed that Orthodox priests learn basic medicine during their theological training and that they assume medical care of their parishioners in rural areas. Both the Russian and the Swedish attempts to revive clerical medicine failed, in part because the churches feared that practicing medicine would divert priests from their pastoral duties.[49]

Enlightenment medicine was learned medicine for university-trained elites, who had studied theoretical medicine, while a broad spectrum of nonelite forms of healing existed for the poor. They included treatment by self-taught surgeons, barber surgeons, apothecaries (who often served as general practitioners), bonesetters, cataract couchers, and unlicensed nonprofessional healers, who often knew some theoretical medicine.[50] Although Galenic medicine was no longer taught in university faculties of medicine, many physicians continued to use it. In Catholic countries traditional forms of religious and folk healing, some of it sanctioned by the church, much of it merely tolerated, continued to exist. However, because of the secularizing tendencies of the new science, it is probable that the use of magic and religious healing had decreased by the seventeenth century.[51]

But time and place were variable factors. In Protestant countries, too, various kinds of folk healers worked alongside licensed and unlicensed medical practitioners. Magical healing was found among those who thought that spells, amulets, and incantations were efficacious. In many cases the line between folk healing and magical practices was blurred. Herbal lore may have represented empirical remedies or magic, as in the case of traditional treatments for warts. Doubtless they were understood differently by different people. As in every culture quacks abounded, the superstitious turned to occult practices, and unorthodox healers gained sensational reputations.[52] Perhaps the best-known unorthodox healer on the Continent was Franz Anton Mesmer (1734–1815), who acquired a following with his controversial demonstrations of "animal magnetism," a precursor to hypnosis, which attracted large numbers of patients and was even supported by the Berlin Academy. Mesmer's ideas were secular in nature, and his healings consisted in shifting the patient's attentions away from consciousness toward an "inner sensibility of the body," which anticipated later New Age mind-body therapies.[53]

The Doctor at the Bedside

The eighteenth century marks the last century of prescientific medicine. While there were many learned practitioners in Europe and America, and while knowledge of the body in certain fields, especially anatomy and physiology, was widely increased, conventional healing made little use of it. Much of it dealt with theory and was not closely connected to clinical training or therapy. Its real contributions to health and medicine lay not in therapeutics but in the belief that governments ought to play an active role in regulating or controlling health, medicine, sanitation, and the environment and its encouragement of conquering disease and lengthening human life.

In the late seventeenth century, Hippocratic medicine, which went back to Thomas Sydenham in the 1670s and was based on classical ideas of humoralism and environmental factors in disease, such as weather and bad air, once more gained popularity among practicing physicians. It was eclectic and without a general theory of nature to replace those of Galen and Avicenna, but it emphasized the "Hippocratic" methods of close observation and use of reason, together with skepticism regarding the use of medical intervention, relying instead on the healing power of nature. Physicians returned to holistic medicine, whose treatment consisted in creating regimens for individual patients rather than giving the same treatment to a group of patients who suffered from the same disease.

Although Galenism had lost its dominance in medical thought, Galenic therapeutics continued to be widely used until the early nineteenth century. The traditional recourse to purging and phlebotomy, based on a Galenic model that viewed sickness as caused by a buildup up of humors that needed to be discharged regularly, remained unabated. The prominent eighteenth-century American physician Benjamin Rush recommended bloodletting for virtually all ills. Other common procedures were bonesetting, plasters, and amputations. Nevertheless, plagues such as bubonic plague and smallpox, which had afflicted Europe and the New World for centuries, declined after 1800, the latter because of inoculation. But syphilis, called the "great pox" or the "French disease," which appeared for the first time in the early sixteenth century, continued to be widespread. Infectious and epidemic diseases over which medicine was helpless—diphtheria, measles, influenza, and gastro-intestinal infections—remained the prevalent killers for another century, especially among the young. By the end of the nineteenth century, with sanitary reforms and a better diet, as well as improved living conditions, epidemic diseases fell off markedly.

Life expectancy was greater for those living in the country than for those living in the poor, overcrowded sections of many cities. Nearly all therapy was non-institutional, administered by physicians or other healers. Most primary care occurred in the home, administered by one's family members, usually by women. Country women possessed knowledge of medical lore that had been passed down for generations. They often produced drugs in their homes, especially herbal remedies, and kept personal journals of new or traditional cures. Well-to-do and aristocratic women sometimes helped the sick poor. In villages without physicians the local clergyman provided learned medicine, while wise women administered folk remedies. Most infants were delivered by midwives. The physician, when called, could often do little more than relieve symptoms, while surgery was limited to a few procedures (removal of fistulas, bladder stones, and cataracts) because there were no effective anesthetics and no way to prevent infection.[54]

While physicians had a large supply of drugs available as powders, ointments (of which mercury was common), salves, and syrups, they were a mixture of ancient and modern, some efficacious and some drawn from folk medicine or alchemy. Some of both kinds were known and used as early as the time of Dioscorides (first century AD) and Galen. Astrology and natural magic were common to both learned and popular practitioners, and in some cases their methods of treatment were not very different. It was difficult to diagnose the causes of most diseases, since they were as yet unknown. The patient's urine was tested, and temperature and pulse were taken. In conducting physical examinations, the doctor depended largely on his five senses.[55]

Much illness, whether treated or not, was healed by nature, as it always had been. Many conditions were not healed; indeed, those suffering from them did not expect them to be healed, but hoped for some relief and were grateful for any they received. The compassion, care, and sympathy found in one's family went a long way toward providing a sense of security and gratitude. Death came, usually in the home (except among the sick poor), surrounded by family and often with a clergyman at the bedside. The knowledge that the time and circumstances of their leaving the world, like that of their coming into it, was in God's hands brought a comfort that is often lacking in our own day. Today we expect our lives to be prolonged and death to be delayed, pain to be alleviated, disease cured, and physical comfort restored. In the premodern period life was simpler, therapeutic resources were limited, the sick had fewer expectations, pain was a normal and concomitant aspect of both sickness and therapy and accepted stoically, while medical treatment remained much the same as it had been since ancient times.

Chapter Eight

The Nineteenth and Twentieth Centuries

Anglo-Saxon Protestantism, which provided the backdrop to so much of North American life and culture, was deeply influenced by the Evangelical Revival, which was spread in the mid-eighteenth century by the preaching of John Wesley and George Whitefield (1714–1770). A series of revivals in the American colonies between about 1730 and 1760 (the First Great Awakening) has traditionally been credited with the evangelical spirit that would permeate virtually all denominations of American Protestantism.[1] Later revivals in America, between c. 1800 and 1830, are called the Second Great Awakening. The spread of the revivals to the frontier resulted in the planting of new churches, and by midcentury evangelicalism was dominant in most American denominations, especially among Baptists and Methodists. It gave impetus to a number of social movements, including temperance, prison reform, abolitionism, and poor relief.[2]

Reformation Protestants had stressed philanthropic and humanitarian activity less than Roman Catholics did. Although the issue sometimes provoked tension, many of the well-known humanitarian efforts of the nineteenth century stemmed from evangelical influences in Britain and America, which created a tradition of voluntary charitable activity that continues today. Perhaps the chief motive for humanitarian work was evangelistic, but a concern for human souls sometimes led to a desire to relieve the suffering and poverty of those to whom evangelicals ministered. This compassion resulted in charitable work on behalf of prisoners, prostitutes, deprived children, and the poor generally. It also provided a stimulus to active campaigning for humanitarian legislation, particularly in England, where evangelicals such as William Wilberforce (1759–1833) and the Earl of Shaftesbury (1801–1885) led movements for factory and prison reform and for the abolition of the slave trade. But they preferred to deal with social problems by voluntary charity, believing that aid by the state could never duplicate the compassion and concern for individuals and their souls that motivated private philanthropic efforts.

The Origins of Modern Nursing

The impetus for the extensive philanthropic hospital care in Catholic countries was provided by Catholic nursing orders. However, the tradition was largely lacking in Protestant churches until the nineteenth century. In the eighteenth and nineteenth centuries, Britain relied on voluntary organizations to support hospitals. Churches did not fund hospitals but encouraged Christians to donate to hospital charity. Hospital Sunday was created by some British churches to encourage their parishioners to contribute to the support of voluntary hospitals.[3]

The founding of Protestant nursing orders was chiefly the work of Pastor Theodor Fliedner (1800–1864) and his wife, Friederike, who created the Deaconesses' Institute in Kaiserswerth, Prussia, in 1836. Fliedner, pastor of a small Lutheran congregation, traveled extensively to raise funds for his struggling congregation. On his journeys he observed the many benevolent hospitals in Holland and England, which often had better buildings than nursing staffs, and they inspired him to found an institution that would meet the need for nursing care of sick and neglected children. He was influenced by the philanthropic and evangelistic work of the Quaker prison reformer Elizabeth Fry, but he borrowed the idea of deaconesses from Mennonites in Holland. Pietists in Germany had already begun to work toward the creation of a nursing order of Protestants similar to those in Catholic countries.

A practical man, Fliedner recognized the paramount need for trained women and founded a school to train them. He established the Order of Deaconesses in 1836, the same year that he founded the Kaiserswerth Deaconesses' Institute, which graduated its first deaconess two years later. The institute trained three classes of deaconesses: those who cared for the sick and poor as well as those in asylums; those who planned to teach; and those who assisted in parish work. They wore no habit or distinctive dress but were trained in biblical knowledge so that they could provide spiritual as well as medical care. Soon they could be found all over Europe and in several foreign countries. Fliedner's travels abroad resulted in the spread of nursing orders to other Protestant denominations. On visits to England and Scotland he was influential in the decision of both the Church of England and the Church of Scotland to found nursing homes operated by deaconesses. At the time of his death more than four hundred deaconesses had been trained at Kaiserswerth and related institutions.

The first Catholic hospitals in America were established in the eighteenth century in New Orleans and other heavily Catholic Gulf Coast cities.[4] Catholic sisters also staffed the Baltimore Infirmary in the early 1820s. In 1828 the Catholic Daughters of St. Vincent founded a hospital in Saint Louis, and in 1849 a young Lutheran pastor, William A. Passavant, began a deaconess hospital in Pittsburgh. They became models for private hospitals that American churches began to establish. By the mid-twentieth century, religious foundations accounted for one out of six American hospitals. The number of Catholic hospitals declined in the latter third of the twentieth century because the church had called nursing orders to broader forms of ministry beyond Catholic institutions and because there was a sharp decline in the number of sisters available to staff these institutions in the 1970s and 1980s.

Fliedner's best-known pupil was Florence Nightingale (1820–1910).[5] Her interest in nursing led her to visit several hospitals before traveling to Paris to study the system of nursing of the Sisters of Charity of St. Vincent de Paul. In 1851 she spent several months in training at Kaiserswerth. In 1854, during the Crimean War, she volunteered to raise a nursing staff to care for wounded English soldiers in the Crimea. Having arrived just after the battle of Balaclava, she found the English hospitals in Scutari filthy and badly neglected, reflecting the general deterioration of English hospitals by the nineteenth century. Nurses were untrained, often without any education, and popularly regarded as low-level workers who drank too much because of the easily available alcohol in hospitals and were sexually active because of the number of young men in training, who took advantage of them.

Florence Nightingale gave dedicated service to the English wounded in spite of having contracted fever herself, and her staff reduced the death rate from 40 percent to 2 percent. Her deep personal devotion and her stellar accomplishments in the Crimea brought her much recognition on her return to England, but her health was severely impaired and she temporarily retired. A popular subscription was raised in her honor to establish the Nightingale Training School for the training of nurses at St. Thomas's and King's College Hospitals in 1860. Although Nightingale remained in poor health, she was consulted by foreign governments during the American Civil War (1861–65) and the Franco-German War (1870–71) regarding nursing and hospital care. She worked for sanitary reform in the Indian army, as well as among Indians and the poor generally, emphasizing the importance of cleanliness, especially in homes. Against much early opposition and male prejudice, Florence Nightingale, by her personal character and sheer persistence, inaugurated a new era in caring for patients.

Asylums for the Insane

The nineteenth century saw a change in public attitudes toward mental illness and its treatment. Probably no other kind of illness has suffered from so much misconception, from theories of demonic possession to the view that those who suffered from mental illness were criminals who had to be kept confined in chains. The most famous asylum for the confinement of the insane in England was the Bethlem Royal Hospital in London. Originating as a priory in 1247, it became a hospital in 1337 and began admitting mentally ill patients in 1357. It was notorious for the inhumane treatment of its inmates; those who were considered dangerous were manacled and chained to the wall or the floor. Bedlam, as it became known, gave its name to the confusion and uproar that in the public imagination characterized conditions in an asylum. The asylum was relocated several times, but as late as the early nineteenth century it retained its reputation for poor treatment of the inmates by an uncaring staff. Such treatment, while common throughout Europe and America, was not found everywhere.[6]

In Paris in 1793, Philippe Pinel (1745–1826) came under political suspicion when he sought permission from the revolutionary Paris Commune to free from their chains some mentally ill patients in the Bicêtre Hospital.[7] His *Traité medico-philosophique sur l'alienation mentale* advocated a more humane treatment. Early attempts to provide humanitarian treatment of the insane in England were made by two English Quaker philanthropists. One was William Tuke (1732–1822), a tea merchant who followed in a family philanthropic tradition that was characteristic of the Friends. After a Quaker patient died under mysterious circumstances in the York County Asylum, Tuke suggested that the Friends might create an institution for their coreligionists who suffered from mental diseases. In 1796 he opened the York Retreat, an asylum that cared for thirty patients in a supportive family setting. Tuke may have been influenced by another Quaker, Dr. Edward Long Fox, who, after operating a small private asylum, in 1804 built a new asylum in Brislington, near Bristol, to house seventy patients. It became a model institution for its treatment of the insane. The patients had no restrictions; they were encouraged to spend time outdoors and to participate in useful work in the upkeep of the building and grounds. Fox had probably been influenced by Pinel during his several trips to Paris. His treatment consisted in hypnosis and mesmerism (the latter was fashionable at the time).

The philanthropic efforts of Tuke and Fox attracted public attention and led to the demand for reform of the poor conditions then prevailing in public asylums like Bedlam. The findings of several select committees of the House of Commons led to the eventual abolition of mechanical restraint in favor of seclusion.[8] Interest in the causes of mental illness led to a decline in views that insanity was God's punishment for a dissolute life, and they gave way to physical explanations. But insanity continued to be popularly attributed to moral as well as physical factors, including masturbation and intemperance.

Medical Missions

European colonial powers were not initially interested in providing medical services to the general populations of colonial possessions.[9] Their focus was primarily on protecting Europeans (administrators and settlers), and they were concerned particularly with efforts to eliminate the causes of epidemic diseases. Hence it fell to missionaries to provide clinics and hospitals for colonial subjects at the local level. Given their dedication to medical philanthropy through nursing orders, it is not surprising that Catholics pioneered medical missions. Missionary activity was carried on chiefly through evangelistic orders such as the Jesuits, but they were complemented by nursing orders. As early as the sixteenth century the Jesuits had established more than 150 hospitals in Mexico alone.[10]

Among Protestants, medical missions did not begin to play an important role in missionary activity until the second half of the nineteenth century. Two missionary doctors, Peter Parker (1804–1888) and David Livingstone (1813–1873), pioneered Protestant medical missions. Parker, an American Presbyterian doctor and minister, was the first medical missionary to China. Sent by the American Board of Commissioners for Foreign Missions in 1834, he opened an eye hospital in Canton the next year. It was the first Christian hospital in the Far East. Livingstone was a Scot who experienced an evangelical conversion at age seventeen. Born into a poor family, he saved enough to study medicine and theology before going to Africa in 1841. He became the best-known missionary of his day, and his explorations of Africa made him a household name throughout the world. More than any other person, he was responsible for making slavery illegal throughout the civilized world. Protestant missionaries brought European moralistic ideas of bodily hygiene and sanitation, which were often undertaken with crusading zeal and formed a key element in Protestant approaches to medicine. Many missionaries who had no medical training undertook rudimentary medical work, which they considered an effective prelude to evangelism and a necessary component of compassionate concern for local needs.

Medical missions developed slowly at first. One estimate put the number of European medical missionaries in 1852 at a mere thirteen. Mission societies feared that medical work would interfere with the primary goal of missions, which was the salvation of souls. This attitude gradually underwent reevaluation as mission societies came to recognize medicine as a desirable and even necessary part of missionary activity. At first, Protestants thought of it as mainly strategic, a means of gaining a hearing for Christianity in areas where mission work did not find ready acceptance. In fact, the conversion rate among patients in mission hospitals was extremely low. According to Ronald Numbers and Ronald Sawyer, "During one twelve-year period the Medical Missionary Society of Canton treated more than 400,000 patients but managed to convert only a dozen of them to Christianity."[11] Not only did patients interpret their healing in Christian hospitals in the light of their own religious beliefs but the missionaries did not integrate their religious teachings into medical healing. This attitude gave way by the end of the century to the view that the alleviation of human suffering was a Christian duty that reflected the compassion Christ demonstrated by his healing the sick.

Protestants came to view medical missionary endeavors as a practical manifestation of the gospel, undertaken in obedience to Christ's commands, and not merely a means for the conversion of souls. Over time, medical missions tended to abandon efforts to use medicine in the service of evangelism and were content to make medical service an end in itself. Nevertheless, in China the number of medical missionaries had risen to 650 by the end of the nineteenth century, and more than one-third of American mission stations in China carried on medical work. Beginning in the 1860s, women began to undertake medical work, especially among Chinese women, in a strategy that became known as "Woman's Work for Woman."[12] As a result, women increasingly undertook training in medicine, some of them as physicians once medical schools began to admit women students in the late nineteenth century.

In the nineteenth century, missionaries were expected to perform many tasks. The primacy of evangelical work created some tension among members of the medical staff, who believed that their training and dedication to healing had equipped them primarily for medical work. In the twentieth century, medical professionalism and the secularization of medicine resulted in medical missionaries' devoting themselves exclusively to medicine. As mission hospitals and clinics became more scientific, their religious role was diminished. By the 1950s and 1960s, as most colonial territories became independent states, they often viewed missionaries with suspicion, as agents of Western neocolonialism. By the 1970s many hospitals founded by missionaries had either closed for lack of personnel or been taken over by newly independent governments. Nationals replaced missionaries, and many hospitals that had been founded by missionaries no longer had any on their staffs. By the end of the twentieth century it appeared that the era of Western medical missions was nearing its end.[13]

No element of Catholic philanthropy in America has been as impressive as the organization of medical care by nursing orders of nuns.[14] The earliest nursing sisters offered mostly palliative care, but they were quick to learn new techniques, and the discipline of the orders provided good training for the founding and administration of hospitals and other medical institutions. The most famous Catholic institution for the care of the sick in America is St. Mary's Hospital in Rochester, Minnesota. On August 21, 1882, a tornado struck Rochester, a town of five thousand, creating much devastation and leaving thirty-one dead and hundreds injured. Mother Alfred Moes, a Franciscan nun who had come to America from Luxembourg in 1851, initially to help Native Americans, and the Sisters of Saint Francis of Our Lady of Lourdes, an order that she had founded in 1877, worked with a local physician, Dr. William Worrall Mayo, to assist the injured.

Mother Alfred later approached Dr. Mayo with the idea of creating a hospital that would serve Rochester. He had founded the Mayo Clinic with his sons, Drs. William J. and Charles H. Mayo, in 1887. An Episcopalian, Dr. Mayo initially saw difficulties with the proposal, but Mother Alfred responded, "The cause of suffering humanity knows no religion or sex; the charity of the Sisters of St. Francis is as broad as their religion."[15] She promised that her order would raise the necessary funds. After delays caused by prior construction commitments, St. Mary's Hospital opened in 1889 with a staff of five nursing sisters and room for thirty-five patients. Under the determined leadership of Mother Alfred, the hospital grew to become the largest privately operated hospital in America.

The success enjoyed by Catholic nursing orders in the New World was unparalleled and testified to the vision of the sisters to serve a philanthropic mission that was especially characteristic of the Franciscans, who excelled in medical charity. But it also reflected the desire to use medicine in the service of saving the souls of patients, as well as the Catholic emphasis on the necessity of good works to one's salvation. By the Second Vatican Council, in the 1960s, nursing orders of nuns had created 950 Catholic hospitals in the United States, with 156,000 beds that served 16 million patients a year. In addition, they had founded 376 homes for the elderly and 337 nursing schools. This growth occurred during the era before the rise of the feminist movement and constitutes an enormous accomplishment for Catholic religious orders of women.[16]

Diverse Approaches to Health and Healing

The nineteenth century saw the rapid naturalization of medical theory as the specific causes of disease were discovered within a matter of a few decades. Belief in God's direct and immediate involvement in human sickness had long before begun to diminish, even in the minds of the religious, with the rise of rational-speculative medical theories. But it persisted into modern times as a means of accounting for epidemics, for which there were no explanations that could be readily translated into prevention or cure.

Throughout history, Christians, like people of all faiths, often viewed outbreaks of plague as God's providential judgment. Once the causes of a disease had been discovered, however, Christians ceased to use theological explanations. That was true of smallpox in the eighteenth century, following the widespread use of inoculation, and of cholera and diphtheria in the nineteenth century. When pandemic outbreaks of cholera occurred in the first half of the nineteenth century (in 1832 and 1849), they provoked the same theological responses that earlier epidemics had drawn. Repentance and moral reformation were seen as the only preventive. But by the 1860s, John Snow, a London physician, had convincingly traced the cause of cholera to contaminated water supplies and demonstrated that improved sanitation was the only effective preventive, though whether he influenced American practice is not clear. But during the next decade, the germ theory of disease stimulated bacteriologists to search for microbial causes of most diseases, including those that were epidemic.[17]

Health and healing concerns were never central to Protestant Christianity. Unlike Catholic belief and practice, traditional Protestantism had no place for the encouragement of contemporary miracles—no healing shrines, no appeal in prayer to saints for healing, no sacramental rites of healing. With the exception of some post-Reformation movements, Protestants historically looked to medicine for healing or relief from pain, and the physician enjoyed an honored position in Protestant communities. It was largely through the Holiness movement that faith healing came to prominence in pietistic circles in the late nineteenth century in both European and American Protestantism. Traditional Protestants held that miracles had ceased with the close of the apostolic age at the end of the first century. Miracles accompanied revelation, and when revelation ceased, miracles did as well. Protestants acknowledged that God sometimes healed in answer to prayer and without medical means. But they considered supernatural healing to be an occasional and special manifestation of God's providence (God's activity in the natural order), and they distinguished it from faith healing.

On both sides of the Atlantic, Protestantism experienced a surge of interest in religious healing in the late 1870s that resulted in a number of new healing movements.[18] Some prominent Pietist preachers in Europe, such as Christoph Blumhardt in Germany and Otto Stockmayer in Switzerland, attracted adherents by their ministries of healing. In America, among those who sought to reclaim for the church a ministry of healing that they believed had played a significant role in apostolic times were several evangelicals. The most notable were A. B. Simpson (1844–1919), founder of the Christian and Missionary Alliance, and A. J. Gordon (1836–1895), a nationally prominent Baptist minister in Boston. Both came to believe in faith healing after experiencing personal healing themselves. In *The Ministry of Healing* (1882), Gordon, appealing to Jesus's commands to his disciples to heal (e.g., in Mk 16:15–18) and to the Christian belief in the unchanging nature of God and his world, argued that miraculous healing was a privilege that was intended for Christians of all ages and therefore ought to enjoy a permanent place in the ministry of the church. But he warned against making healing an end in itself and deprecated fanaticism in the matter.

Simpson came under the influence of Dr. Charles Cullis, a former Boston physician who maintained an influential ministry of religious healing, and Simpson's belief in faith healing was partly responsible for his decision to leave the Presbyterian ministry for an independent one. In *The Gospel of Healing* (1877), Simpson went much further than Gordon. He argued that in his death on the cross Jesus bore both human sin and sickness. Hence the Christian believer could claim divine healing apart from physicians and medicine because it was always God's will to heal. Late in his ministry, Simpson gave less prominence to faith healing and refused to support the sensational healing campaigns that were held in America by the Australian faith healer John Alexander Dowie (1847–1907), which attracted wide attention. Dowie, who was known for his hostility to physicians and medicine of any sort, created a healing center at Zion City, Illinois, that attracted seven thousand people, many of whom claimed to have been healed.

The Prayer-Gauge Debate

During the early 1870s a controversy arose in Britain over whether belief in miracles was credible.[19] The protagonists were James B. Mozley, a theologian and later Regius Professor of Divinity at Oxford, and John Tyndall, a distinguished physicist. The issue of whether miracles violated the principle of the uniformity of nature had been raised by Baden Powell in *Essays and Reviews* (1860), a volume that challenged traditional views of supernatural revelation. Powell argued that the inductive principle was the basis of science and that it demonstrated the uniformity of nature and left no gaps to be filled by miracles. In his Bampton lectures (1865), Mozley asserted, in response to Powell, that the principle of the uniformity of nature did not preclude belief in miracles, because natural laws were descriptive, not prescriptive. John Tyndall argued in reply that induction was the basis of science, and cause and effect a universal principle that had never been disproved.[20] Empirical research—observation and experiment—was the means by which science advanced and its theories were tested. With the knowledge of science expanding, miracles might someday find explanation in natural causes. Tyndall went on to question "special providences" as well. Special providences were God's activity in nature, such as answers to prayer, which were viewed as providential though not miraculous by the eye of faith. Tyndall placed such a view of divine activity in the same category as miracles, magic, and witchcraft that were part of an anachronistic world-view.

The controversy led to Tyndall's questioning the efficacy of petitionary prayer. In 1872 he proposed a scientific experiment along the lines suggested by Sir Henry Thompson, a prominent surgeon. To discover whether prayers for the sick were efficacious, Sir Henry had recommended that one hospital ward be set aside for patients suffering from diseases whose mortality rates were known and that for a period of three to five years they be made the object of special prayers. They would be supervised by "first rate physicians and surgeons." Their mortality rates would then be compared with those of patients who had not been prayed for but had been treated medically. Hence Sir Henry pitted medical science against religion in obtaining physical healing. The proposal became known as the "prayer-gauge." Tyndall was confident that the trial would demonstrate the superiority of the "scientific" method over spiritual healing.

The debate drew distinguished partisans from all sides. They included such distinguished personages as James McCosh, president of Princeton, a Scottish Presbyterian, and Francis Galton, Darwin's cousin and the founder of eugenics. It provoked ingenious arguments and much fine rhetoric. While the trial was never undertaken, the gulf that its proponents believed existed between scientific naturalism and the religious world was challenged by the discovery that the mind had the ability to affect the healing of the body and by a new interest in spiritism and psychical research by a number of leading scientists and philosophers, such as William James and Alfred Russel Wallace, the codiscoverer of evolution by natural selection. While these views did not necessarily lead to belief in a God who heals, they helped to bridge the gap between the two sides. By the end of the century a conflict between a scientific understanding of the world and belief in God's activity in it no longer seemed as clear cut as it had in the 1870s, and research into mysticism and psychical research seemed to offer promise for finding connections between the spiritual and material worlds.[21] At the same time, the Prayer-Gauge debate signaled major tensions in the relationship between science and religion that developed in the late Victorian period, in large part because of the controversy over the publication of Charles Darwin's *The Origin of Species* (1859).

Biblical Criticism, Evolution, and the Professionalization of Medicine

Two radical developments in nineteenth-century Protestantism that struck at the roots of supernatural religion, namely, biblical criticism and Darwinism, were to have long-term significance for medicine. Biblical criticism, which began in France and Germany in the eighteenth century, was based on naturalistic assumptions that were derived from the Enlightenment. Christians had always held the Bible to be the product of God's revelation to humankind, written by prophets and apostles under the influence of divine inspiration. Proponents of the new criticism viewed it as a fully human product and studied it as they would any ordinary ancient text, rejecting such supernatural elements as prophecy and miracles. They assumed as well evolutionary theories of the origin and development of religion as a natural phenomenon. Religious consciousness as depicted in the Old and New Testaments, they asserted, was culturally conditioned, reflecting the limitations of time and place.

The new biblical criticism, which was often called "higher criticism," was initially introduced into American universities and seminaries in the late nineteenth century by professors who had studied in Germany. Conservative Protestants rejected these views as incompatible with supernatural Christianity. Others (many mainstream Protestants and theological liberals) incorporated them into their thinking and attempted to redefine Christianity by retaining only those elements that could be accommodated to the new "scientific" thinking.[22] For theological liberals, religious experience rather than special revelation as found in the Bible became the basis for redefining faith and morals. They regarded elements of biblical morality as culturally specific, outdated, and no longer normative for modern society. From the late nineteenth century, American Protestantism would be characterized by a theological and moral pluralism, with a range of positions that reflected divergent moral perspectives, some only tangentially related to biblical norms.

Evolutionary theory, even more than biblical criticism, undercut the religious basis of Western societies. This was true not only because of its influence on ideas of the origin of the world and of humanity but also because it challenged historical Christian belief about God's interaction with creation. Although many Christians accepted some form of evolution (usually as theistic evolution), the opposition to Darwin's theory that arose in some religious circles encouraged a polarizing public image of evolution as the chief battleground between science and religion. One of the most influential events in this regard was the celebrated debate, seven months after the publication of *The Origin of Species*, between Samuel Wilberforce, bishop of Oxford, and Thomas Henry Huxley (1825–1895), who was called "Darwin's Bulldog" for his spirited defense of evolution in pseudo-religious terms. The debate came to epitomize the shift in society from privileging religion to privileging science.

While Darwin's theory did not make a significant contribution to clinical medicine, many physicians became advocates of evolutionary naturalism, in which they had no recourse to God or to divine interaction with nature. Early examples were Huxley, who was a physician, and the influential French surgeon and anthropologist Pierre Paul Broca. By the end of the nineteenth century some form of evolution was accepted by most members of the scientific community, resulting in the evolutionary world picture that was to characterize science in the twentieth century. The widespread adoption by physicians of evolutionary naturalism as a world-view was a factor in divorcing medicine from traditional religious ideas and creating a new image of medicine as a scientific enterprise. Perhaps its greatest influence on medicine, however, was that it professionalized science and recast society as one that specifically privileged scientific enquiry.

The professionalization of medicine in the late nineteenth century followed that of other scientific disciplines, such as geology and biology, which had begun earlier in the century. In geology, for example, nonclerical practitioners sought to displace clerical naturalists, who held many of the university positions in the field. In doing so they dropped all theological references (e.g., those relating to natural theology) from their published work in a professionalizing strategy designed to allow them to replace "amateur" clerical geologists in the field. The new strategy encouraged in the scientific professions a spirit of secularism and a weakening of the traditionally close relationship between science and religion, especially in natural theology. The medical profession gradually became secularized as well. With the growing dominance of positivistic science, medicine became more a science and less an art.[23]

In 1910 the Flexner Report, commissioned by the Carnegie Foundation, recommended that American medical schools raise their standards of admission and graduation and that they include additional science in the curriculum. As a result of the report, many small proprietary medical schools were closed and the science curriculum of those remaining was strengthened. As medical schools began to demand of their students a rigorous training in science and to devote their attention increasingly to research, medicine insisted on autonomy and distanced itself from Christian motives of compassion and calling, although Catholic, Baptist, and Adventist medical schools (among others) continued to maintain a Christian model of healing. As a result of the professionalization of medicine, the traditional Christian framework in Protestant, especially Anglo-Saxon, countries diminished in influence with every succeeding generation of physicians.

At the same time, hospitals were undergoing reconstitution.[24] Since their beginning in the fourth century, hospitals had been institutions primarily for the poor. They had given less attention to medical treatment than to relieving individual suffering. Caring for patients, rather than curing them, had been the main element in hospital treatment. Between 1700 and 1850 medical practice improved, and the emphasis shifted from care to treatment and cure. Between 1870 and 1910 hospitals were transformed into centers of medical research and education. Until the last three decades of the nineteenth century the medical care that one could receive from a physician in the home was considered superior to that received in a hospital. Advances in medicine and medical technology rapidly made the hospital a medical necessity, not merely for the indigent but for all seriously sick persons. The professionalization of nursing and the introduction of antiseptic surgery during this period led to a vast improvement in the cleanliness of hospitals and helped to increase their number. As late as 1873 the United States had only 178 hospitals, including mental institutions, with fewer than 50,000 beds. By 1909 the number had jumped to 4,359 with 421,065 beds; and by 1939 to 6,991 hospitals with 1,186,262 beds. Reorganized as businesses rather than charities, they were no longer governed for the most part by nursing orders and religious authorities, but by professional administrators and physicians. As they came to focus on scientific medicine administered under a corporate business model, the model of compassionate and spiritual care, historically the chief focus of hospitals, diminished.

Temperance Movements and Innovative American Religions

Health and temperance concerns were topics of growing interest in American Protestantism in the late nineteenth century. Sanitary reform was endorsed by religiously motivated sanitarians, such as John H. Griscom, who saw the relationship between filth and disease as a moral issue. Griscom was a Quaker physician who sought to improve the health of the lower classes. "Cleanliness," he wrote, "is said to be 'next to godliness,' and if, after admitting this, we reflect that cleanliness cannot exist without ventilation, we must then look upon the latter as not only a moral but religious duty."[25] The influence of Methodism on the evangelical revivals of the eighteenth and nineteenth centuries in England and America led to the growth of temperance movements, as evangelicals sought to promote personal holiness by proscribing the use of such addictive substances as tobacco and alcohol. The movements were supported by ministers and humanitarians and given early medical support by the prominent American physician Benjamin Rush, whose *Inquiry into the Effects of Ardent Spirits on the Human Mind and Body* (1784) became influential.

In 1826, under the leadership of the eminent minister Lyman Beecher, the American Society for the Promotion of Temperance was established in Boston. The movement divided in 1836 over whether temperance required total abstinence but grew in its influence in the first half of the nineteenth century. In 1851 Maine became the first state to forbid liquor sales, and within five years thirteen northern states followed suit. The Women's Christian Temperance Union, formed in 1874, was preceded by the entry of the National Prohibition Party into elections in 1869. The movement gained the support of several (but not all) American Protestant denominations. Presbyterians, while supporting temperance movements in general, rejected calls for total abstinence, while Methodist and Holiness groups supported them. A leading group in favor was the Board of Prohibition and Morals of the Methodist Church.

A growing revulsion against public drunkenness in the last two decades of the nineteenth century resulted in temperance's gaining the support of many American progressives as an issue of social reform. Anti-Catholicism and the fear of immigrants also became factors in the encouragement of temperance movements, which culminated in 1919 in the passage of the Eighteenth Amendment to the U.S. Constitution, which prohibited the "manufacture, sale or transportation" of alcoholic beverages. Prohibition was justified on the grounds that excessive or unrestrained consumption of alcohol led to personal and social evils, such as domestic violence and crimes against women, public drunkenness, and numerous health-related problems. While the temperance movement declined dramatically after the repeal of the Eighteenth Amendment in 1933, large numbers of evangelical and liberal Protestants continued to practice and advocate total abstinence from alcohol, smoking, and addictive drugs.

Traditional Protestantism, with its insistence on an educated clergy and its high regard for medicine, tended to support medical orthodoxy, while several innovative and marginally Protestant American sects aligned themselves, at least initially, with sectarian medicine, which they found more compatible with their medical doctrines.[26] Thus many homeopaths were attracted to Swedenborgianism for its mysticism and its belief in the spiritual harmony of body and soul.[27] Seventh-day Adventism, founded by Ellen G. White (1827–1915), placed great emphasis on the care of the body. Adventists abstained from eating foods that were prohibited in the Old Testament, such as pork and shellfish. In the beginning they were opposed to the use of physicians altogether and advocated religious healing by anointing. But after the death of an Adventist sister who had refused medical assistance, White labeled her stance "fanaticism" and began to support the use of medicine. After a vision in 1863, White undertook an extensive program of health reform that she incorporated into the Adventist belief system. She adopted vegetarianism, hydropathy, and abstinence from tobacco and alcohol, changing her views frequently on what was and was not permitted.[28]

The organization of a health-reform institute was followed by other Adventist sanitariums and medical colleges. Over time the Adventists' emphasis on the healing power of prayer gave way to greater reliance on the skill of physicians. By the mid-twentieth century Adventists' interest in health had caused many adherents to enter the health-care professions, and Adventist hospitals earned a good reputation as health-care centers.

Jehovah's Witnesses, initially founded in 1881 as the Zion Watch Tower Bible and Tract Society, did not focus on health-related issues, but the editor of the denominational magazine *Awake!*, Clayton J. Woodworth, often attacked the medical profession, as well as the use of aspirin and vaccination. Witnesses later attracted attention for their refusal to accept blood transfusions, which the society officially condemned in 1945 as incompatible with the teaching of biblical passages such as Genesis 9:4, Leviticus 17:13–14, and Acts 15:29.[29]

A third religious denomination, Christian Science, was founded by Mary Baker Eddy (1821–1910), who claimed, as had Ellen G. White, divine revelation for the views that she expressed in *Science and Health, With a Key to the Scripture* (1875).[30] Eddy taught that the material world was unreal since there was no reality except that of mind or spirit. She rejected medical healing altogether, holding that disease and death were merely illusions. Christian Science healers sought to persuade patients that sickness did not exist.[31] Nor did they believe in death, which they considered only as "passing." The group had a good deal of influence in the late nineteenth century and even attracted a considerable number of Jewish converts.[32]

A fourth American religious movement that arose in the nineteenth century was the Church of Jesus Christ of Latter-day Saints (LDS), popularly known as Mormonism. It was founded in upstate New York in 1830 by Joseph Smith (1805–1844), who claimed new doctrines that he alleged God had revealed to him on golden plates, which became the Book of Mormon. The new revelations, several of which became separate scriptures, led to many doctrinal innovations, including belief in the plurality of gods, the potential for men to become gods, and polygamy. Following the murder of Joseph Smith, the leadership of the movement fell to Brigham Young (1801–1877), who led a group of Mormons from their colony at Nauvoo, Illinois, to Great Salt Lake in Utah, where he established a Mormon theocracy. The church abandoned plural marriages in 1890. The LDS Church grew rapidly in the twentieth century, spread throughout the world by Mormon missionaries. It was efficiently organized and governed in a hierarchical fashion by the Twelve Apostles of the church in Salt Lake City.

Like other novel American religious movements, the Mormons adopted health measures that were the subject of revelation—the Word of Wisdom—which included the prohibition of stimulants like alcohol and tobacco, the gift of healing, belief in exorcism, and healing by anointing. In their formative years Mormon pioneers practiced medical self-help and valued recreation for its contribution to health.[33] Prohibition of stimulants was relaxed for a time, but after 1900 abstinence from alcohol, tobacco, coffee, and tea became mandatory. In the 1870s Mormons adopted orthodox medicine, which quickly replaced botanical (folk) medicine, and routinely relied on physicians. Although the LDS community eventually accepted conventional medicine, it long distrusted psychiatry, as did many conservative Protestants, but the church established regional networks of professional psychologists for counseling.[34] Throughout the twentieth century it accepted modern medicine in all its forms and avoided taking a public stand on controversial issues in medical ethics, preferring to leave these issues to the personal accountability of its members.

The alternative medicine advocated by these American religious movements was vigorously attacked by traditional Protestants of all denominations, most prominently by the redoubtable Princeton theologian B. B. Warfield (1851–1921) in his *Counterfeit Miracles*. Published in 1918, after the heyday of evangelical faith healing and the origins of sectarian American religious movements that challenged conventional medicine, it had a greater influence than any other work did on subsequent evangelical thinking about the theology and practice of faith healing. It represented a scholarly restatement of the traditional Protestant view that the age of miracles had passed.

Warfield argued that the function of miracles was to accompany divine revelation and to authenticate messengers of God (prophets and apostles). In successive chapters dealing with apostolic healing, medieval miracles, Christian Science, and mind cure, he suggested that faith healing of all types was susceptible of natural rather than supernatural explanation and that it cured only functional disorders and not organic diseases. He distinguished between supernatural healing in answer to prayer, which all Christians believed in, and the expectation of faith healers that God would heal apart from medicine by the exercise of faith alone.[35] Warfield's learning and authority made it likely that mainstream Protestantism would continue to remain within the orbit of orthodox medicine, while alternative healing practices and faith healing would hover on the sectarian fringe of both medicine and Protestantism.

The Fundamentalist-Modernist Controversy and Eugenics

Within mainstream Protestantism, theological liberalism entered the twentieth century as a growing and increasingly dominant force. It adopted late nineteenth-century intellectual currents from Europe, particularly biblical criticism and evolutionary naturalism.[36] By World War I the new thinking had become dominant in most influential American colleges and seminaries. Opposition to modernism (as theological liberalism had come to be called) culminated in the fundamentalist-modernist controversy of the 1920s. The term *fundamentalism*, a neologism coined in 1920, was widely used to describe the beliefs of those who subscribed to the basic tenets of evangelical orthodoxy.[37]

Fundamentalists were unsuccessful in stopping the advance of modernism in the large denominations, most of which became either theologically inclusive or excluded entirely those of orthodox views from denominational leadership and seminaries. Although many conservatives remained within the mainline denominations even while losing their influence, others withdrew into smaller, separatist denominations and independent churches and founded their own seminaries and Bible colleges, as well as journals, mission boards, and benevolent agencies. The victory of the liberals, together with the fundamentalists' creation of new, separatist denominations in the 1920s and 1930s, lessened the visibility and influence of the latter group for a generation, while allowing them to refocus their energy on developing the infrastructure required to support their views. In the 1950s a new generation of leaders, such as William F. (Billy) Graham (b. 1918), emerged, and fundamentalists (or evangelicals, as they preferred to call themselves, after the name historically applied to the evangelical movement in the Church of England) by the 1970s displayed an aggressive, self-confident spirit and made themselves a national force socially and politically.

Some liberals were inclined to adopt novel approaches found in alternative medicine, such as psychic healing, electric energy, yoga, Japanese Reiki (an energy-based healing touch), and elements of Native American animistic spirituality, in place of traditional Christian modes of religious healing.[38] No longer seeking the eternal salvation of human souls, liberals sought to build the kingdom of God on earth through social and political structures. Major Protestant denominations undertook to promote a progressive social agenda and to issue official statements on leading social and political questions of the day.

One of the most notable social issues was the eugenics movement, which sought to improve the human race by eliminating mental illness, retardation, and criminal behavior through such means as compulsory sterilization and restrictions on marriage. In the early decades of the century, the movement attracted broad scientific and medical support in Europe and North America and the approval of well-known Protestant liberals and some evangelicals. Progressive ministers lobbied for legislation to require eugenic sterilization. The findings of research by biologists and social scientists were used to argue that restricting reproduction by those who were mentally unfit would cut welfare costs and reduce social ills. Many American states, Canadian provinces, and countries in northern Europe adopted restrictive measures on marriage.

Liberal ministers, prominent preachers like Harry Emerson Fosdick (1878–1969) among them, advocated selective breeding and eugenic solutions for many of the social problems in America in the 1920s. Religious bodies and leading clergy in England and on the Continent supported national eugenics movements. British scientific and religious authorities formed an alliance to press for the support of eugenics legislation, especially the Mental Deficiency Bill, which was passed by Parliament in 1912. In 1930 Pope Pius XI, in an encyclical on marriage, condemned eugenics. His condemnation was criticized by many scientists and liberal clergy who believed that scientific research supported eugenics. Roman Catholic and conservative Protestant opposition helped to defeat eugenics laws in several states in which the Catholic population was large. In the American South, where fundamentalism was strong, opposition existed but was not as effective, though the passage of eugenics legislation came late, and even the revelation of Nazi eugenic practices after World War II did not wholly discredit it. But there was never a predictable division between Protestant conservatives and liberals over the issue, and one could find individuals from both groups supporting eugenics legislation. Eugenics continues to flourish in the present day in another form, called "genetic engineering."[39]

Pentecostalism and Catholic Healing

With rationalistic attacks on orthodox theology very much a part of the late nineteenth-century intellectual climate, some Christians desired a more vivid manifestation of supernatural Christianity than orthodox Protestantism offered. At the turn of the twentieth century a new movement, Pentecostalism, offered just such assurance.[40] Rooted in the healing movements that arose in nineteenth-century Holiness traditions, it went beyond them in claiming that Christians should seek divine healing instead of medical assistance for all health problems. It claimed that the supernatural gifts of the Holy Spirit described in 1 Corinthians 12 and Mark 16:17–18 were intended to be normative for Christians in every age. The movement originated in 1901 with Charles Fox Parham, a faith healer, in Kansas. His teachings were carried by an African American Holiness minister, William J. Seymour, to Los Angeles, where they led to the Azusa Street revival in 1906, which is widely regarded as the beginning of Pentecostalism in America.

Pentecostalism grew rapidly in the first two decades of the twentieth century. Its distinctive doctrines were the baptism of the Holy Spirit, which it claimed was invariably accompanied by manifestations of miraculous healing and glossolalia, spontaneous speech in a language other than one's own. Pentecostals claimed that they were experiencing a revival of the "signs and wonders" that they believed to be a feature of the apostolic church. They described themselves as proclaiming the "full gospel," by which they meant a restoration of the complete message of New Testament Christianity. Their frequent emotional excesses and bursts of ecstatic behavior caused them to be popularly called "holy rollers." The movement spread to northern Europe, including Scandinavian countries, Britain, and Germany, before World War I. From Europe it was carried to India, and from America to Latin America, where it experienced explosive growth after World War II. By the end of the twentieth century it had become one of the largest Christian movements in Latin America. It attracted many adherents among African Americans, who organized their own Pentecostal denominations in an era characterized by separate African American denominations.

Pentecostals taught that Jesus's death on the cross atoned not only for sin but for disease as well. Hence Christians could claim supernatural healing as a result of offering the "prayer of faith." Pentecostalism produced itinerant healers who claimed that they possessed the gift of miraculous healing, with some practicing exorcism, since they regarded demons as a frequent cause of illness. Several "deliverance evangelists," such as Oral Roberts (1918–2009), were celebrity healers who led highly successful ministries and gained enormous influence in the early 1950s through their weekly television programs, which lasted for some two decades. A focus on demonic possession or oppression by disease, mental illness, and assorted physical ills has remained a continuing feature of many Pentecostal healers. Women pastors and healers were a characteristic element of Pentecostalism during an age in which nearly all Protestant denominations ordained only male clergy. The most famous was Amee Semple McPherson (1890–1944), a colorful performer, media celebrity, and founder of the International Church of the Foursquare Gospel, which became a sizable denomination. Her church, the Angelus Temple in Los Angeles, maintained a "crutch room," where abandoned medical devices could be displayed as material testimony to their healing.[41]

Most Pentecostals rejected medicine in favor of religious healing, believing that God had unconditionally promised to heal, and they attributed any inability to heal either to personal unbelief or insufficient faith on the part of the sick. Some taught that Holy Spirit–filled believers would never experience illness. In the latter half of the twentieth century some Pentecostals modified their categorical rejection of medicine. A minority of Pentecostals came to recognize physicians and medicine as an alternative to supernatural healing, albeit an inferior one. By the 1970s, however, as the movement accommodated itself to American cultural mores and increasingly appealed to an upwardly mobile following, many Pentecostals no longer refused to seek medicine or the care of physicians. Some

Pentecostal ministries established clinics, such as drug-rehabilitation centers, and counseling practices that featured both clinical medicine and prayer.

In 1977 the most famous of the deliverance healers, Oral Roberts, claimed to have had a vision of a nine-hundred-foot-tall Jesus, who instructed him to build a medical center.[42] The City of Faith Medical and Research Center, a major clinic with a hospital, research laboratories, and a medical school, opened four years later in Tulsa, Oklahoma, where Roberts had already founded a university in 1963. The center marked a major transition for the faith-healing minister, who sought to merge prayer and medicine into a holistic view of health. But in 1989, after operating for only eight years, the center closed.

In the 1960s, Pentecostal influences, without a Pentecostal cultural and sectarian flavor, began to infiltrate mainstream Protestant and even Roman Catholic churches. The "Charismatic renewal," as it came to be called, gained widespread influence by introducing religious healing, sometimes of a sacramental nature, to churches that had not traditionally practiced it, especially liturgical churches, such as Episcopal, Lutheran, and Catholic churches in the United States and Anglican churches in Britain and the Commonwealth.[43] An influential early leader of the movement in America was Dennis Bennett, an Episcopal priest, who had experienced the baptism of the Holy Spirit in 1960. Charismatics, as they became known, claimed to have received the "filling," or baptism of the Holy Spirit, and they remained a minority within their denominations, not always enjoying the approval of denominational leaders. In nearly every mainline denomination, however, fellowships of Charismatics were organized.

In the Catholic Church the Charismatic renewal grew out of a retreat held in 1967 for students and faculty members of Duquesne University in Pittsburgh. The movement soon spread to Notre Dame in Indiana and was endorsed by Léo Joseph Cardinal Suenens, a Belgian who was active in ecumenical relations. He was later appointed a papal delegate to the broader Charismatic renewal movement. In the 1970s several Catholic Charismatic priests in the United States developed ministries of healing through prayer, which spread widely throughout Catholic parishes. The Catholic Charismatic movement was received cautiously by the hierarchy but came to enjoy support from Popes Paul VI, John Paul II, and Benedict XVI. In 1990 it was recognized as an ecclesial movement. So quickly did Pentecostalism spread in its many forms that by the year 2000 more than a quarter of the world's 2 billion Christians, both Protestant and Catholic, identified themselves as Pentecostals or Charismatics.

Supernatural healing had always been a feature of popular Roman Catholic piety. It was found most notably at healing shrines, which remained outside the control of the institutional structure of the church. While some Catholics might consider certain manifestations of religious enthusiasm, especially those associated with syncretistic pagan survivals, as superstitious, they reflected an important aspect of Catholic life. There was within the church a tendency, which was not limited to post-Tridentine Catholicism, to blur the distinction between ecclesiastically sanctioned rites and folk practices. The approved observance of venerating relics and blessing animals, for example, seemed to some Catholics not very different from popular cults' attribution of healing or the shedding of tears to statues of the Virgin Mary.[44] Hence there remained within the larger confines of the church as much a place for religious healing as there was within Pentecostalism.

One of the most popular forms was the miraculous healing offered at pilgrimage sites. Beginning in the nineteenth century, Lourdes in France, Fatima in Portugal, and Guadalupe in Mexico have drawn large numbers of pilgrims year after year even though revolutionary advances in medicine were taking place to which they might have looked for scientific medical treatment. But for many pilgrims, medicine could not offer the same emotional or spiritual appeal as the heightened supernaturalism they found at healing sites. Popular Catholic enthusiasm for healing miracles was sometimes focused on living saints, to whom healings were popularly credited. One such saint was Padre Pio (1887–1968), a stigmatic who was alleged to have received in his body the stigmata, or wounds, suffered by Christ in his passion. Padre Pio gained an enormous reputation in Italy for several miraculous cures attributed to him. Miracles of healing continued to play an important role in the process that led to the canonization of saints.[45] But seeking miraculous healing was not the only way in which Catholics approached illness. In addition to those who took part in popular practices that sought divine healing, others, who eschewed publicity, viewed sickness as an opportunity to embrace their own suffering for divine ends, a tradition that dates back to the ascetics of the early church.[46]

Judaism

Modern Judaism is marked by a wide variety of approaches to the interpretation of the Torah (the Law of Moses). Orthodox Jews take a literal approach to the Torah and its traditional interpretation. Conservative Jews believe that the Torah developed historically rather than as absolute divine revelation and that it may be freely adapted to the requirements of modern life. The Reform and Reconstructionist movements take a much more liberal approach to the Torah. They do not consider it to be authoritative or binding except as individuals personally choose to consult it in making moral decisions.[47] There is in modern Judaism no agreed-upon set of doctrines but rather a common group of sacred practices that constitute a core that is accepted by all four branches.

For nearly two millennia the primacy of the Talmudic tradition has been central to Judaism. The Talmud comprises the Mishnah (oral interpretations of the Torah by rabbis) and the Gemara (rabbinic discussions of the Mishnah), which was compiled between CE c. 200 and c. 500. Together they form a cumulative tradition of Halakha, the body of legal rulings intended to make the Torah apply to everyday life. In Judaism the Torah has been viewed through the prism of collections of rabbis' responses or answers to queries regarding its interpretation. These responses do not present straightforward answers to complex issues. A long history of rabbinic discussion has resulted in a great diversity of opinions when applied to any issue, including those that fall under the modern rubric of medical ethics.[48] Because Halakhic discourse takes place within the covenant community, some modern Talmudic scholars have stated that their responses are intended only for Jews, while others have incorporated a broader basis of moral reasoning that constitutes a Jewish perspective in contemporary discussions of medical ethics. Some, such as Immanuel (later Lord) Jakobovits (1921–1999), one-time Chief Rabbi of the United Kingdom, have argued for their applicability to modern philosophical bioethics.[49]

Although a number of Talmudic texts deal with medicine or physicians, many more have to do with the duty of every Jew to visit the sick within the Jewish community. For many Jews, the concept of *tikkun olam* (lit., "to repair [or perfect] the world") means that Jews are responsible not only for creating a model society among themselves but for undertaking the welfare of society at large. This concept has encouraged the Jewish community to assume compassionate, educative, and societal roles that provide healing for the larger world. It has provided the basis for medical philanthropy in the establishment of hospitals, clinics, and medical research. In the twentieth century, Jews have been prominent in the medical professions to a degree that is far beyond the comparatively small size of their faith community within Western societies that are overwhelmingly Christian or secular.

The Hospice Movement, Hospital Chaplains, and Faith Community Nurses

With the majority of people in Western industrialized countries in the twentieth century living much longer than their parents and grandparents did, dying became medicalized, as increasing numbers dealt with "end-of-life" issues. By the end of the century it was not uncommon for patients to die in hospitals, surrounded by high-tech equipment, or isolated in nursing homes. And while everything was done to make the passing of life painless and comfortable, the patient was frequently under sedation. The family often was not present, the physician visited only briefly, and institutional care had replaced the home and the family. Bedside care had become increasingly depersonalized, and the patient seldom knew the physician or nurse well, if at all. In the 1960s, the medicalization of dying attracted a good deal of unfavorable attention from researchers and the public. Elizabeth Kübler-Ross, among others, argued that death and dying had become a social problem and that the dying were too often dehumanized, isolated, and mistreated by the medical system that cared for them.

As concern grew in the last third of the twentieth century among both healthcare professionals and their patients, a variety of attempts were made to introduce changes. The most successful was Hospice, a modern movement that has deep historical roots, which sought to free the dying from medical treatment that merely prolonged life after it had ceased to be meaningful and to normalize the process of dying by placing the person in familiar surroundings, with palliative care that provided comfort at the end of life.[50]

The modern Hospice movement owes much to Cicely Saunders (1918–2005), an English qualified nurse who conceived the idea of helping the dying as the result of an evangelical conversion to Christianity at the age of twenty-seven. Saunders became a nurse, earned a BA from Oxford, and qualified as a medical social worker, later working in several hospices, including St. Luke's, a hospice for the dying poor. In 1951 she began further medical studies and obtained her medical degree in 1957. On June 24, 1959, while she was reading her daily devotions, the idea of founding a hospice for the dying came to her. It was, she said, inspired by her reading of Psalm 37:5: "Commit thy way unto the Lord; trust also in him; and he shall bring it to pass." Eleven years later she was able to establish a hospice-care institution, St. Christopher's, where she sought to emphasize concern for the spiritual, social, and psychological well-being, as well as for the physical pain, of patients approaching death. Saunders traveled internationally to advocate her ideas, and she influenced Florence Wald, dean of the Yale School of Nursing, who had worked with Saunders in England, to found the Hospice movement in America in 1971. Since then the movement has spread to nearly every country in the world. In 2009 it was estimated that there were ten thousand programs that had been created with the purpose of providing palliative care to the dying.

In the United States, Hospice began as a volunteer movement, but it soon was covered by health insurance. Today Hospice care is largely delivered in homes, though it is also available in health-care institutions of all kinds. It is covered by Medicare and has become so widely used that in 2008 more than one-third of Americans in the last stages of illness were dying in the their homes under Hospice care. In Canada, by contrast, hospice care has been administered in hospital settings, although only two provinces provide insurance coverage for the service. In 2004, 5–15 percent of Canadians benefited from the program. In Britain, hospice services are provided both in traditional hospices and in the home.

With the secularization of health care in the latter half of the twentieth century, faith communities became increasingly peripheral to bringing spiritual counseling to hospital patients. This phenomenon reflected the tendency of Western societies to move away from organized religion to an individual expression of spirituality. To fill the void, hospital chaplains, some part time, some full time, were added to the professional staffs of most hospitals and mental-health institutions. Originally they were drawn from mainstream Protestant and Catholic traditions, but as immigration brought patients from a variety of non-Christian backgrounds, the religious pool of chaplains was enlarged. Over time, pastoral care has come increasingly to be administered by hospital chaplains rather than by religious communities. In the pluralistic religious culture that replaced the traditional Christian one in the late twentieth century, chaplains were expected to minister to believers and unbelievers alike, to Sikhs, Hindus, Muslims, and secularists as well as to Christians and Jews. With the rapid growth of hospital chaplaincy as a profession, a professional chaplaincy association was formed in 1946 that has established uniform standards for certification and standards of practice.[51]

Modern nursing practice in Western countries has largely been based on the model of Florence Nightingale, who viewed nursing as a vocational calling that mingled compassionate care of the sick with spiritual nurture. As health care became secularized, both in hospital and private nursing, an attempt to bring spiritual concerns into health care was the creation of faith community nursing (FCN), also known as parish (or pastoral or congregational) nursing. The movement owes its inspiration to the nineteenth-century Lutheran deaconess movement, in which nursing was seen as a vocation. FCN was founded in the 1970s by a Lutheran pastor, the Reverend Granger Westberg, who was involved in holistic healing centers that sought to integrate pastoral care with medical care. Westberg advocated a team approach to health care, with nurses constituting the vital

link in bringing the church to patient care. He developed a model in which parish nurses were associated with congregational ministry to the sick. The movement has spread to broader ecumenical and interfaith movements, where local
congregations minister to their parishioners in their illness. They also emphasize
disease prevention and community health as a component of the church's calling
to minister to the whole person. In the United States alone there are some twelve
thousand FCNs, and the movement has spread to other countries.[52]

Roman Catholic Medical Ethics

Beginning in the Middle Ages, moral theologians in the Western (later Roman
Catholic) Church created and modified over time a highly intricate system of
ethics based on canon law, that is, authoritative rules that the church imposes in
matters of faith and morals. Since the Council of Trent there has been a strong
Catholic emphasis on the natural-law tradition, which views God's intended
purposes as evident in every human act. The principle of double effect, which
was formally defined by Jean Pierre Gury in the nineteenth century, occasioned
much discussion among medical ethicists in the twentieth century. It addresses
the question whether one can ever do evil to achieve good. Some actions produce effects that produce both intentional good and unintentional evil. Can such
actions be justified? Is there a way to justify exceptions to absolute moral prohibitions?[53]

Any human intervention that affects the way a person functions naturally is
subject to the application of the principle of double effect. In the area of medical
ethics it has focused on issues at the beginning and end of life, such as contraception, abortion, artificial insemination, and euthanasia. But it has made contributions to larger areas of medical ethics as well. One is the principle of totality,
according to which it is licit to harm one part of a human organism for the sake
of the larger whole (a principle used, for example, to justify organ donations). A
second is the distinction between ordinary and extraordinary means as a way to
decide when it is acceptable to discontinue life support.[54]

The Catholic Church has banned all forms of artificial contraception, although
the prohibition has been contested in the tradition.[55] The Catholic tradition long
emphasized that procreation was the primary purpose of the sexual act, with
other purposes viewed as secondary. In 1963, Pope John XXIII created a commission that he charged with examining overpopulation, a charge that he later
extended to include the specific issue of artificial birth control. The commission completed its recommendations, which it delivered to a new pontiff, Paul

VI, in 1966. Two years later, in 1968, Pope Paul issued an encyclical, *Humanae vitae*, in which he announced that given the divided opinions of the commission, he intended to restate the traditional teaching of the church regarding artificial contraception as well as sterilization and abortion. Because the tradition had regarded the natural intent of sexual intercourse as being to conceive children, the artificial prevention of conception was unnatural and therefore sinful. Hence the encyclical prohibited all means of artificial birth control. *Humanae vitae* first made the explicit statement that there exists an inseparable connection between the unitive and procreative purposes of sexual expression in marriage. It also confirmed the Catholic acceptance of the rhythm method as a means of natural birth control. The encyclical uses such language as "recourse to infertile periods" and "responsible parenthood." In so doing it suggests the church's acceptance of married couples' choosing to have fewer children, although each specific sexual act must remain open to the possibility of pregnancy.[56]

In spite of Pope Paul's hope that the encyclical would be accepted by Catholics, it was attacked from both inside and outside the church. Paul VI, according to Marvin O'Connell, "provoked the most severe crisis of authority within the church since the Reformation." "No papal teaching document has ever caused such an earthquake in the Church," wrote Bernard Häring. "Reactions around the world—in the Italian and American press, for example— are just as sharp as they were at the time of the Syllabus of Errors of Pius IX [1864], perhaps sharper."[57] The pope was accused of having fallen under the influence of the conservative minority of the commission. Some moral theologians stated that view openly, and several left the church. The crisis pitted what had become modern cultural norms against the authoritative teaching of the church. As a result of the conflicting claims of contemporary culture and religious authority, *Humanae vitae* produced a crisis of conscience for many married Catholics. It encouraged what came to be called "cafeteria Catholicism," the practice of selectively choosing to accept some but not all Catholic teaching.[58] While the practice was not new among Catholics, the term emerged among orthodox Catholics to indicate that the church's teaching on sexuality was not a negotiable issue but one that was central to the tradition.

Protestant Medical Ethics

While Roman Catholics could claim a long tradition of reflection and writing on issues in medical ethics, the first major modern attempt to treat the subject systematically by a Protestant was *Morals and Medicine* (1954), by Joseph

Fletcher (1905–1991), based on his Lowell lectures, delivered at Harvard in 1949. Fletcher, a theologically liberal Episcopalian, broke new ground in basing medical ethics, including issues such as the use of contraceptives, artificial insemination, sterilization, and euthanasia, on the patient's right to decide what should be done rather than on specific biblical or Christian principles. Initially, Fletcher became interested in the way technology allowed for expanding choice in these areas. He would later attract attention for his formulation of "situation ethics." Rejecting absolutist ethics, he maintained that nothing was wrong in itself and that the agent's ethical intention should be based solely on love.

Very different from Fletcher's approach was that of the Methodist Paul Ramsey (1913–1988) in *The Patient as Person* (1969). Ramsey too focused on the concept of patients' rights, but Ramsey's more traditional theological stance placed both physicians and patients within a context of covenant fidelity.[59] Fletcher and Ramsey assumed that the patient was a free and autonomous moral agent, an assumption that was to become axiomatic to the discussion of medical ethics by Protestant, and indeed nearly all, medical ethicists in the last third of the twentieth century. Both men were concerned with the role of agape, God's self-giving love. Fletcher argued that it was enacted through the will without moral rules, and Ramsey that it was "inprincipled," or enshrined in rules that were based on divine revelation and required obedience.

Concern for patients' rights reflected the spirit of the age, which sought greater individual freedom in every sphere of life, and fit neatly into the culture of American individualism. It stressed personal freedom and choice but differed from the Enlightenment concept of human autonomy in being constrained by the rule of love and one's accountability to God. Physicians' paternalistic attitudes toward patients came to be regarded not merely as anachronistic but as an affront to patients' freedom to be informed, to choose which procedure was best, and to control their destiny. Justifying the proliferation of patients' rights required a good deal of legerdemain on the part of Protestants, since the biblical tradition emphasized the sovereignty of God, absolute norms within a moral framework (such as that of the Decalogue), limitations on human freedom (in such matters as ending one's life), and the sanctifying value of suffering. Hence ethicists like William F. May preferred to speak from a perspective of covenantal responsibilities rather than from one of patients' rights.[60] Issues in medical ethics increasingly split Protestants along the fault line of a liberal-conservative divide, with liberals like Fletcher arguing from a consequentialist or personalist perspective that veered toward relativism, and conservatives like

Ramsey and May arguing from a more traditionally biblical and deontological view based on covenant partnership.

The differing Protestant approaches were especially apparent in the case of divisive issues like abortion and euthanasia. Attitudes toward both reflected distinctively Protestant perspectives on questions of moral theology. While neither abortion nor euthanasia was specifically condemned in scripture, both seemed contrary to the spirit of several biblical passages and had been almost universally condemned by Christian moral theologians since the second century AD.[61] Conservative Protestants believed that abortion was incompatible with the doctrine of the *imago Dei* (image of God), according to which God had created the human race in his likeness.[62]

Yet, in the matter of abortion, as with suicide, the issue was not as clearly defined as it was in Catholic moral theology. Some Protestants argued that extenuating circumstances (e.g., danger to the life of the mother) might sometimes justify abortion on the ground that an actual life was of greater value than a potential one. Others believed that additional, if exceptional, instances (e.g., rape) might justify abortion. Hence there was within the Protestant tradition some willingness to recognize exceptions to the general prohibition of abortion.[63] Nevertheless, Protestantism was characterized by a strong pronatal position. With the sexual revolution of the 1960s and the rapid growth of secular attitudes, there was a growing demand in Western countries for more liberal abortion laws. The controversy became sharper in the United States following the Supreme Court's legalization of abortion in its decision in *Roe v. Wade* (1973).

In the 1980s, the issue of euthanasia came to the forefront, initially over the ability of physicians to extend life artificially through support systems. In the 1990s the debate was broadened to include the legalization of physician-assisted suicide.[64] Liberal and progressive Protestants argued for the freedom of the autonomous individual to end his or her own life. The "right to die" was, they asserted, a personal decision like any other and should not be restricted by law or professional medical constraints. Conservatives were opposed to active, but not necessarily to passive, euthanasia. Most recognized that the development of life-support systems had permanently altered the process of dying and that there were instances in which nothing useful was gained by extending the life of a merely vegetative patient. Evangelicals' firm belief in an afterlife provided support for their position.[65]

But active euthanasia and physician-assisted suicide seemed different. Conservative Protestants argued that God was sovereign, the author of life and death, and that physicians usurped God's prerogative when they assisted a patient in ending his or her own life.[66] By the end of the twentieth century the liberalization of laws in the Netherlands and the United States (beginning in Oregon) suggested that the right to an assisted death would become yet another matter of choice guaranteed by law to patients. In a society that sought to maximize individual rights, it seemed to be merely the logical extension of already existing rights. But attempts to remove legal and social impediments to physician-assisted suicide drew a good deal of opposition from conservative Protestants of many denominations, as well as Roman Catholics, a fact that testified to the continuing strength of traditional Christian moral opposition to suicide and euthanasia.

If abortion and euthanasia provided the most highly visible focal points of tension among Protestants regarding medical-ethical concerns, it was human sexuality that proved to be the most divisive. The traditional Protestant pattern for sexual behavior included well-defined hierarchical gender roles within marriage and abhorrence of those practices that were regarded as directly contrary to God's intended sexual standards (e.g., fornication, adultery, homosexuality, and lesbianism). In the Protestant pattern of companionate marriage, matrimony was a school for character that provided a safe and natural outlet for sex, encouraged the conception of children within a nurturing relationship, and promoted mutual support. Well into the twentieth century most Protestants considered artificial contraception to be immoral, an attitude that doubtless owed something to Victorian attitudes toward sex as well as to the secular and humanist origins of the family-planning movement.

The immorality of artificial contraception was defended partly by appeal to scripture (Gen. 8:8–10 was sometimes cited) and partly by the argument that it was inconsistent with a belief in divine providence and that it encouraged promiscuity. In 1930 the Church of England became the first Protestant communion officially to accept the morality of birth control, and other Protestant bodies and theologians followed suit. Acceptance, which was widespread by midcentury, was made easier for Protestants than for Catholics by the conviction that intercourse existed for conjugal pleasure as well as for procreation. In the last third of the century, owing to a neo-Malthusian concern about overpopulation and its effects on the standard of living throughout the world, theological liberals argued that couples and nations had a moral responsibility to limit their populations in order to preserve scarce resources. Conservatives, on the other hand, emphasized the personal moral issues inherent in the use of contraceptives, particularly that it might encourage promiscuous sexual activity.

The legalization of abortion by the Supreme Court's decision in *Roe v. Wade* divided Protestants as perhaps no other issue had since the fundamentalist-modernist controversy of the 1920s. It galvanized pro- and antiabortion support-ers (the former preferred to define their position as "pro-choice"), who organized pressure and lobbying groups. One of the defining issues in the culture wars of the last third of the twentieth century was what came to be called "family values," a term coined by the Moral Majority. The term was shorthand for a complex of moral questions that included limiting sex to marriage, opposition to abortion and euthanasia (the "right to life"), and considering homosexual practice a per-verted form of sex. Almost invariably, mainline Protestant denominations, which were dominated by theological liberals, advocated open views toward sexual and reproductive issues (under the banner of the right of a woman to control her own body), while conservative Protestants defended family values. Although Catho-lics approached the issues from a different and older stream of moral theology, they often sympathized with the coalition of like-minded Christians and others who held traditional views toward sex.

During the same period, new technologies (e.g., medical experimentation on human subjects, artificial insemination, in vitro fertilization, organ trans-plantation, cloning, and stem-cell research) raised a number of ethical issues, forcing ethicists of all points of view to define their positions. Not surprisingly, the response among Protestants has lacked a general consensus.[67] On the one hand, with their longstanding adherence to the Baconian premise that scientific knowledge leads to human progress, Protestants have been inclined to welcome the application of technology to medicine. On the other hand, they are a diverse people, divided into many denominational (and nondenominational) commu-nions and reluctant to accept any single interpretation of highly complex issues.

In a number of medical-ethical issues there has been no single Protestant po-sition. One cannot look to official pronouncements of denominations for author-itative statements, since they frequently represent the views of a small group of theological or ethical professionals that are unrepresentative of either the main-stream clergy or the lay members of the larger communion. And the very fact that Protestant denominations issue position statements has seemed for many clergy and laymen to be contrary to the tradition of Protestant voluntarism and indeed an attempt to impose a particular point of view that inhibits the exercise of private conscience.[68]

No single person or group within Protestantism can be said to speak for the church. The Protestant emphasis on subjection to the word of God in scripture has led to what Paul Tillich called the "Protestant principle," the refusal to absolutize the relative, whether it is found in human traditions or in ecclesiastical institutions and pronouncements. And while Protestants have remained divided over the validity of Enlightenment-based higher criticism of the Bible, which enjoyed unquestioning acceptance within liberal Protestant circles during the twentieth century but was generally rejected by evangelicals and other theological conservatives because of its anti-supernaturalist assumptions, they were reluctant to disregard biblical injunctions, especially on moral issues. As a group, Protestants have tended not to be as concerned with complex issues raised by modern medical technology, which appeared to be well understood only by specialists, as they have been about matters of personal morality, which have influenced them more directly. And on moral issues laymen have been hesitant to abandon traditional interpretations of scripture, often being more conservative than their clergy.

On one issue, however, that of genetic engineering, initially there was widespread (though by no means unanimous) agreement across the theological spectrum. Several Protestant writers on biotechnology suggested caution in genetic experimentation, exhorting researchers to avoid usurping God's role. Some American Protestant denominations issued pronouncements expressing approval of genetic research but warned against genetic engineering. Protestants of all persuasions opposed the patenting of genetic material. But differences existed. Conservatives opposed the use of prenatal genetic screening on the ground that it encouraged abortion. A deeper concern for conservatives, such as Gilbert Meilaender, who gained prominence because of his writing and testimony on cloning and stem-cell research for the National Bioethics Advisory Commission, was that transgenic animal research and human cloning might alter the genetic makeup of humans and lessen their distinctiveness as a unique species created in God's image.

The issue here was bound up with the definition of the *imago Dei*. Was it determined by genetic makeup or defined in terms of such factors as rationality or a spiritual and moral sense? On the other hand, theologians like Ronald Cole-Turner, in *The New Genesis* (1993) and *Human Cloning* (1997), and Ted Peters, in *Playing God?* (1997), argued that humans were "created co-creators" with God through biotechnology and that genetic engineering offered the potential for a partnership with him in an ongoing work of shaping and directing creation, which remained open to human exploration and manipulation.

The debates over biotechnology revealed a clash between Baconian optimism and the recognition that there was a potential for harm arising from original sin and human pride. Both are traditional Protestant motifs. But the debates also invoked the Christian theme, by no means exclusively Protestant, of humans' stewardship over nature, involving the care of creation that God entrusted to the human race, with a special concern for other creatures. Keith Thomas found in this tradition of care for the environment, which extends in the English Dissenting tradition from the Puritans to John Wesley, the intellectual origins of later campaigns against cruelty to animals and indeed of stewardship of the earth.[69]

Secularization and Alternative Healing

During much of the twentieth century Western medicine no longer had formal ties to a religious culture. No appeal was made to spiritual values in medical treatment except among a minority of health-care providers who themselves felt a vocational calling. Spiritual values were diminished or eliminated as the influence of traditional religion in medicine declined. Hospitals and charitable medical facilities became secularized as well, with the decline of Catholic religious orders and the transition of faith-based hospitals to community-based or for-profit corporations. Mainstream medical ethicists in the last three decades of the twentieth century adopted secular consequentialist perspectives in place of implicitly religious ones even in religious educational institutions and hospitals with formal religious connections.[70]

Concurrent with the abandonment of traditional religious ties in American public life has been the widespread following accorded New Age spirituality that developed in the later half of the twentieth century with the goal of creating an expanded spiritual awareness.[71] The movement drew on Eastern pantheistic religions and metaphysical traditions, as well as naturopathy, mesmerism, spiritualism, anthroposophy, and theosophy, which appealed to the newly fashionable motifs of religious inclusivism and pluralism. It claimed to merge science (which sometimes appeared to outsiders to be pseudoscience) with an alternative spirituality that sought to create an approach to healing that was holistic, based on natural substances, and vitalistic.[72]

New Age spirituality became popular in the 1960s and continues to attract widespread interest, even if in a diffused and attenuated fashion. Indeed, it might be considered to be a component of the spirit of the age. Because it rejects defined theology and creedal formulations in favor of pantheistic or nonparticularized views, it has coalesced easily with modern secularism and has influenced education and the professions, including medicine. Complementary and alternative medicine (CAM) is very much a component of New Age belief, which rejects "biomedical ethnocentrism" and orthodox or conventional medicine, together with their methodological naturalism, in favor of self-healing and self-realization—the two are often intertwined—which are intended to create a harmony of body, mind, and spirit.

Holistic medicine rejects the naturalistic world-view of biomedicine. It strives to restore harmony between the physical and metaphysical planes of reality. It includes elements of traditional Chinese medicine (TCM), such as t'ai chi, acupuncture, yoga, and herbal remedies, as well as naturopathy, reflexology, aromatherapy, Ayurveda, and various forms of psychic healing.[73] While some of these practices remain marginal in traditional medicine, others, such as yoga and acupuncture, have been incorporated into routine medical practice and mainstream medicine.[74] Additionally, New Age therapies have been adopted by practitioners of holistic medicine. They include crystal healing, therapeutic touch, and other therapies that allegedly channel healing energies into the body from astral and etheric planes.

A growing number of medical clinics offer an integrative medicine that combines alternative medicine with orthodox practice, while a high proportion of American medical schools offer courses in alternative therapies. There is a strong spiritual component in much of CAM, which is variously derived from Hindu or Tibetan roots and Native American or European pagan backgrounds. But it more commonly appears as an amorphous patchwork of folk-healing practices drawn from a wide variety of spiritual sources, rather than traditional religious communities, and is little noticed because it operates outside conventional medicine. It has benefited from a variety of folk and ethnic traditions introduced by recent immigrants to North America from Mexico, the Caribbean, and Southeast Asia. In a sense, CAM resembles nineteenth-century American religious movements that advocated alternative healing. Although it is not affiliated with any religious movements and indeed operates independently of them, its debt to Eastern contemplative and metaphysical traditions has proven to be attractive to many.

The Modern Era

By the end of the twentieth century, the "Protestant empire," which had dominated Anglo-Saxon values for some two centuries, no longer retained its unchallenged position in the formulation of widely accepted societal values. In the latter half of the century it appeared that religion was being pushed to the margins of society. Increasingly divorced from public life, it seemed to be confined largely to the private sphere as the structures of society reflected the pervasive *fin-de-siècle* cultural motifs of pluralism and diversity. The authority of the Catholic Church over many of its adherents had been diminished as contemporary cultural values challenged the moral and theological teachings of the church. Protestant influence was weakened by the virtual disappearance of the once prominent public role that the clergy had played in American public life, together with the decline in their theological and moral authority both inside and outside the churches. The once influential mainline American Protestant denominations had become deeply divided theologically and were embroiled in ongoing disputes regarding faith and practice that made it difficult to arrive at any consensus on controversial issues or even to define core doctrines. Hence Protestants came to have few effective means of enforcing the authority of their churches or formulating theological creeds or moral standards for even their own constituencies.

Many historians of American religion, however, reject narratives of secularization and declension to explain the status of religion in the twentieth century.[75] While appearances suggest a process of secularization in contemporary American society, the historical record supports a more complex story of ever-increasing levels of religious belief and church membership (the opposite of declension, in fact) offset by changes, but not necessarily a diminishment, in the role that religion plays in American life. The distinctively Protestant understanding of the individual and his or her conscience alone before God, together with the Protestant insistence that a Christian's calling must be lived out in the world, has continued to serve as an influential motivating factor in the medical professions.

The Roman Catholic Church has survived controversies over clerical celibacy, the church's prohibition of contraceptives, and other issues of moral theology that grew out of the progressive atmosphere that produced the Second Vatican Council. The ecclesiastical hierarchy has moved gradually but decisively in a conservative direction since the heady days of post–Vatican II liberalization. The centralized structure of the church has equipped it to meet some of its challenges, including the charges in North America and elsewhere of widespread sexual molestation of children by some priests. But although it remains an influential force in moral and medical-ethical debates, its hold over its constituency has been considerably weakened by serious defections. Liberal mainline Protestant denominations have experienced significant losses of members and influence in the past several decades and face what appears to be long-term decline and probable consolidation. But newer churches, many of them attracting recent immigrants, have sprung up in communities across American and European countries that have opened their borders to immigration. Hence the frequently predicted decline of religion as a result of scientific and secular forces in American life appears contradicted by evidence that often escapes public notice.

A new component in the religious mix, Eastern and New Age spirituality, has provided an aura of mystery that fits well with the nonreligious stance of public institutions, particularly educational and medical institutions. It has furnished a vague and nonoffensive vocabulary, such as the use of *spiritual* in place of *religious*, that cloaks the philosophical materialism of some nonreligious or secular assumptions, while allowing the listener or reader to supply whatever construction he or she chooses to give it. Particularly in medicine it has added a note of reverence that might give comfort and a sense of mystery to one confronting issues of sickness and death. It can be equally well adapted to atheism and religious belief.

The future is contingent, and historians make worse prognosticators than do tea-leaf readers. Only time will tell how issues at the intersection of medicine and religion will be resolved in the context of an age in which the traditional monotheistic religions appear comparatively less influential in the Western world. But immigrants have brought into developed countries new movements that, operating outside traditional denominational structures, have created noninstitutional churches. These churches, often built from the ground up, are vibrant in their fellowship and mutual concern. Many of them reflect evangelical or Pentecostal/ Charismatic approaches. The rapid growth of Islam in North America and Europe is too recent to assess, but it is likely that it will become a strong religious movement in the West in the course of the twenty-first century, making contributions to the understanding of health and healing that reflect distinctly Islamic perspectives.

Historians who attempt to understand the present lack the ability to evaluate current trends retrospectively and therefore to assess whether they will prove in the long run to be more than a mere flash in the pan. History is replete with surprises, sudden turns, and wide swings of the pendulum, and it is impossible to predict where the whirligig of fashion in new or recycled ideas, together with new religious movements and popular culture, will carry us. Wherever they do, we are likely to see reappearing in new contexts many of the same themes that were present whenever religion and healing intersected in the past.

Epilogue

Historians today are less likely than they were a generation ago to talk of continuities in history. Contemporary historical discussions of human culture assume that most ideas and practices are culture-specific.[1] Most historians today reject positivism, the belief that by collecting data one can accumulate sufficient evidence for an objective understanding of society and its progress. They eschew as well Whiggism, the assumption that history has moved progressively toward our culturally superior age to create the institutions that exist today. Instead historians view past cultures as distant and many of their ideas as outdated. To speak of common values that transcend societies and temporality is widely regarded today as an attempt to maintain a conceptual unity among human beings that does not exist. Humans, in this reckoning, are bound by the constraints of their own social and economic structures and share little in their outlook and values with earlier societies.

The issue becomes more focused when we consider the differing views throughout history of how the body operates. On the one hand, we have in common with previous generations biological similarities that all humans share in the experience of birth, death, sickness, and pain. On the other hand, we interpret those events through the lens of our medical and cultural understanding. Does our knowledge of bacteria, DNA, and the HIV virus create a wall that prevents us from understanding the medical models of past cultures and peoples?[2] The answer is a complex one, but in spite of differences in culture and world-view that do indeed separate earlier historical societies from our own, one finds even in societies that preceded us by millennia commonalities that allow us to identify their creators as people with whom we have more in common than we have differences.

It may be impossible to understand fully the world-view of an ancient society, just as it is impossible to comprehend fully the world-view of another human being whom we include among our acquaintances. But in the case of our contemporaries, that limitation does not prevent communication across even quite pronounced cultural and linguistic barriers. The fact that we observe artifacts in prehistoric cultures that allow us to reconstruct a civilized society that came into being at the beginning of human history demonstrates that there are recognizable human values that transcend the category of culture-specific. These patterns inform our discussions of comparative cultures, including healing and medical ethics. People in earlier centuries held very different views of health and disease than we do in the twenty-first century. But by emphasizing their differences to the neglect of their similarities, we create an unnecessarily restrictive lens through which to view past medical cultures.

It may indeed be the case that the culture of ancient Greece, to take one example, is, in M. I. Finley's phrase, "desperately foreign." Over time Greek ideas have been transformed, modified, or discarded. Yet we observe characteristic features of Greek society that are recognizable because we have observed them in some form in our own culture. We see in fifth-century BC Greece the origins of a medical tradition that is naturalistic in its approach to healing. We observe the emergence of a medical profession that is recognizable in the subsequent developments of the physician's role. We see in the Hippocratic treatises the earliest attempts to develop professional ethics that we still appeal to in our own century as providing the roots of medical etiquette and professional behavior. "First do no harm" (*primum non nocere*) has become one of the most widely quoted Hippocratic aphorisms,[3] and it forms the basis of the principle of non-malfeasance in medicine today.

Compatibilities of Medicine and Religion

Religion has complemented medicine in similar ways in many cultures and in nearly every age. One way is in attempting to account for suffering in general and sickness in particular. We term these attempts *theodicies*.[4] The Old Testament book of Job gives us the best-known theodicy in the Western tradition and one that is still widely acknowledged for its profound discussion of the purpose of suffering. From the Roman Stoics we read consolatory literature that addresses universal themes in death and dying that are not vitiated by the limitations of Stoic doctrine.

Medical ethics too has been influenced by religious values. Hippocratic medicine, which first formally defined medical ethics, was a professional ethic, rooted in the culture of the medical craftsman rather than in any religious or moral values. In the early Middle Ages the religious and philanthropic ideas of Christianity merged with the earlier secular tradition of Hippocratic ethics. Both came to form important strands in Western medical ethics. The introduction of the Christian emphasis on compassion as an essential motive of the physician represented a fundamentally new ideal. In the latter half of the twentieth century Greek medical ethics gained new attention as a result of a renewed interest in medical ethics, while religious ideals continued to underlie ethical concerns in faith-based medicine and health-care institutions.

Religious views have contributed to theories of disease and its cause and cure. Ancient Near Eastern societies, especially in Mesopotamia and Egypt, believed that disease could be inflicted by demons or by the employment of malignant magic. They depended on a range of healing procedures that included naturalistic remedies, magical incantations, and prayers. The early Hebrews, by contrast, were forbidden by the Torah to employ pagan religious and magical means. Yahweh was the only healer, and he healed through natural processes as well as through prayer or the agency of prophets. In the fifth century BC, the addition of theory to medical practice made it possible to explain disease in terms of natural causation. But side by side with a naturalistic and secular medical tradition, there existed a parallel and complementary tradition of religious medicine in which the sick sought healing directly from the god Asclepius rather than from a physician. Greek naturalistic medicine was taken over without religious scruples by Jews, Christians, and Muslims, who had no objection to a theoretical system that had shed any religious connections it once had. Suni Muslims adopted Greek medicine without its parallel tradition of religious healing, while Shia Muslims supplemented it with a tradition of religious healing. Early Christians accepted natural healing as normative, although they and most Christians in all ages have believed that God can and does on occasion heal apart from medical means.

Greeks and Romans saw in philanthropy a potential motive for the practice of medicine but never believed it to be an essential qualification for the medical practitioner. Classical philanthropy excluded pity as a motive for medical treatment. The larger cultural values of Greco-Roman society also militated against medical philanthropy. They included the Stoic conception of *apatheia* (insensibility to suffering) and a spirit of quietism that regarded attempts to improve the world as fruitless. With rare exceptions, no religious impulses for charity involved personal concern for those who required help. Hence, there were no pre-Christian institutions in the ancient world that offered charitable aid, particularly health care, to those in need.

Yet the ideal physician and the physician as an ideal are types encountered with frequency in classical literature. The word *iatros*, "physician," when used figuratively in Greek literature, is not a neutral term. Unless it is modified by a pejorative adjective, it usually carries with it the metaphorical force of an objective and unselfish man who is dedicated to his responsibilities. Thus the good ruler, legislator, or statesman is sometimes called the physician of the state. Essentially, it was thought, the statesman was (or should be) to the state what the physician was to his patient. We find this symbolism in nonmedical literature as early as the fifth century BC. Similarly, ancient philosophers were frequently described as physicians of the soul. Regardless of whether the "medicine" they administered was soothing or painful, the good of their patients was always their proper object. The Greeks themselves came to expect much of medicine, and of the physician too. The art of medicine itself carried with it a humanitarian expectation quite apart from any externally defined ideal, such as that found, for example, in the deontological literature of the Hippocratic Corpus. And while compassion was not an ideal of medical care, the literature enjoined kindness and sympathy.

It is not surprising, then, that early Christians spoke of Christ as "the Great Physician" (*Christus medicus*). Basic to Christianity was a philanthropic imperative that sought to meet human needs. It was based on agape, the incarnational and redemptive love of God in Jesus, who provided the model for the sacrificial love of one's fellow human beings. Of Jesus's teachings none was to become more influential in this regard than the parable of the Good Samaritan (Lk 10:25–37), with the command, "Go and do likewise" (v. 37). The compassion demonstrated in Jesus's parable was anticipated in Judaism, appearing in such passages as Deuteronomy 22:1–4, where the Torah commands the return of the lost property of a neighbor even at considerable personal cost. It underlies too the account of Israel's liberation of the captives of Judah after their defeat and capture (2 Chron.

28:5–15), which has been termed "a grand archetype of the deed of compassion" described in Jesus's parable.[5]

In the first two centuries of their existence Christian churches were unique in establishing congregational forms of organized assistance for the care of the sick and the poor. The first hospitals resulted from this long tradition of the care of the sick. The best-known, and the earliest, was the Basileias, completed in about 372 by Basil the Great. Hospitals spread rapidly throughout the Eastern Roman Empire, appearing in the Western Empire a generation after they were established in the Greek world. Early hospitals and related institutions grew out of the monastic movement, and the monastic orders provided much of the personnel to staff them.

The first hospitals were founded specifically to provide care for the poor. Until the mid-nineteenth century, hospitals remained what they had been intended to be in the beginning, institutions for the indigent. Diaconal movements and religious nursing orders that provided palliative care constituted another branch of Christian medical care. They have existed in many forms in the history of medical philanthropy. Among the best-known are the medieval Knights Hospitaler; the Sisters of Charity, founded by Saint Vincent de Paul in the seventeenth century; and the Lutheran diaconal movement, founded by Theodore Fliedner in the early nineteenth century.

Beginning in the eighth century, medical philanthropy became a characteristic feature of Islam as well. Like Christianity, Islam emphasized the community's responsibility to those who needed help. While Islamic hospitals were not as widespread, we know of thirty-four in a world that stretched from Spain to India. They were characterized by a high level of medical and administrative skill and had specialized wards, including those for women and for the insane. The belief that good works were necessary for salvation was a motivating factor in Muslim philanthropy. In all the Abrahamic faiths medical philanthropy was rooted in religious concerns.

At the intersection of religion and medicine, one of religion's most significant roles has been to provide consolation in sickness and death. The consolatory literature of a long Christian tradition has brought solace to bereaved family members by urging them to seek help from God and employ spiritual remedies to assuage their loss. Suffering played a positive role in Christian thought that it lacked in classical paganism, which saw in it no redeeming qualities. In Stoicism, sickness was one of those indifferent matters (*adiaphora*) that must be endured. European secular traditions, beginning with Epicureanism, have seen little that was positive in suffering. From the perspective of those who have no expectation of an afterlife, euthanasia was and is a natural and humane solution because it ends interminable and meaningless pain.

By contrast, in the Hebrew Bible, Jews who suffered sought consolation from Yahweh but saw suffering as sometimes coming from the hand of God. Most constructively, painful and chronic disease should not bring self-pity; rather, they should offer the opportunity for drawing near to him. One finds this theme in Job. At the end of his trials, in which he was vindicated by Yahweh, Job could say, "I had heard of you by the hearing of the ear, but now my eye sees you" (Job 42:5). Christianity went further, focusing on suffering as an element that God used for the believer's spiritual benefit. Gregory of Nazianzus attributed a threefold purpose to sickness: purification from sin, a testing of virtue and of one's philosophy, and the provision of examples of patient endurance. The theme was a common one in the writings of the church fathers. Sickness invited self-examination and, when it was found to be the result of sin, the possibility of confession, repentance, and spiritual restoration.

The motif of sickness as chastisement, while a constant theme in spiritual writers, was considered less significant by Christians who viewed illness as the result of the Fall. Illness and disease were the common lot of humanity, and most disease was otherwise unrelated to sin. In Islam, illness was regarded as a test not only for sufferers but also for those, such as children or parents, who looked after them. Suffering taught patience, trust in Allah, and (to caregivers) compassion for the sick. Islam did not emphasize the theme of sickness and death as divine punishment for sin.

"In the midst of life we are in death."[6] The care of the dying was an extension of ministry to the sick. In the fifteenth century a genre of literature grew up that was intended to prepare one for death. A later example, and the best-known in English, is Jeremy Taylor's classic devotional work, *The Rules and Exercises of Holy Dying* (1651). Taylor's treatment of his subject differs from the medieval approach in that he makes the whole of life a preparation for dying. John Wesley, who admired the work, made a practice in his itinerant preaching of visiting jails to offer spiritual counsel to men facing the gallows. It was not only compassion that pastors offered but concern for the souls of those about to die. Were they ready to meet their Maker? If so, the sting of physical pain and death was removed by anticipation of heaven, which would bring release from suffering, the hope of meeting loved ones, and the certainty of seeing the Creator face to face. Of the benefits that religious certainty offered the dying, none was greater than the hope it gave of the life to come.

Tensions in Religion and Medicine

I have argued that medicine has historically enjoyed diverse relationships with religion that have often been complementary and beneficial. But there have been tensions as well. They include the condemnation of medicine by some religious writers; the view that religious healing is superior to reliance on medicine or that it is God's sole intended means of healing; the proscription of certain kinds of medical procedures or treatments; the glorification of disease for spiritual growth; and the attribution of disease to demons, with exorcism the only means of healing.

While it is easy to find denunciations of physicians among such early Christian fathers as Tertullian, most of the early Christian critics of medicine accepted natural healing from physicians, as did Tertullian, who only denounced the use of medicine in cases of abortion and euthanasia but otherwise accepted it gratefully. A handful did not. One who had great reservations was Tatian (fl. second century AD), who rejected the use of drugs, which he believed allowed demons to gain access to the body. He did not, however, altogether oppose the use of medicine. One also finds ascetics in late antiquity who denigrated physicians and claimed the ability to heal supernaturally. In fact, however, their denunciation of physicians was largely rhetorical, designed to support their claims to be able to heal diseases that physicians could not heal.

One can find in every generation a few Christians who rejected medicine altogether. Martin Luther's early colleague in the Protestant Reformation, Carlstadt, believed that Christians should look to God for supernatural healing rather than to physicians. In the late nineteenth century, the Australian faith healer John Alexander Dowie routinely condemned physicians who employed natural remedies, and he founded his own celebrated faith-healing center in Zion City, Illinois. Carlstadt and Dowie, while representative of a certain type of Christian who held hypersupernaturalistic views, were atypical in condemning all medicine. Nevertheless, faith healing came to enjoy considerable popularity in the late nineteenth century among Protestants in America and Europe, and it helped to create the charged atmosphere that gave rise to Pentecostalism in the early twentieth.

While Pentecostalism is only the most recent in a history of healing movements within Christianity, it enlarged and extended the minority belief that for every illness Christians should call on God to heal apart from medical means and in answer to the prayer of faith. Faith healing in the twentieth century produced many independent and itinerant healers, both men and women, who attracted large followings by making sensational claims to be able to heal all diseases. They appealed most naturally to those for whom medicine had been unsuccessful, but they also appealed to sincere believers who expected God to reward their faith by granting them supernatural healing. One finds the appeal in Protestant sectarian faith healers as well as in Catholic shrines. Cases of alleged healing were given much publicity, while little attention was given to the vast majority who were not healed, many of whom were likely to have been disappointed that their faith had not been strong enough to merit healing. For many too their religious faith must have been weakened as the result of their failure to experience healing where the promise was not matched by the result.

But one should not condemn all "healing ministries." Believers have always maintained that God sometimes heals through prayer as well as by means of traditional rites of healing such as anointing. Many pastors and chaplains routinely pray for healing with sick patients and either privately or in small groups administer some form of sacramental healing. They avoid unconditional promises but seek to provide pastoral care and encouragement. Some believe that God has given them a special gift that will benefit those who seek them out, and they cite credible instances of extraordinary healing in their personal ministry. What is dismaying in faith-healing movements is the global claims of some to be able to heal all those who have faith, the sensationalism they foster, their constant appeal for funds, and the marketing and media coverage that some employ, which seems to reflect little concern for the bodies and souls of those they claim to help. Even here, however, the evidence is ambiguous. Some of the sick are helped, even healed, by the most objectionable kinds of faith healers. Does one attribute the healing to supernatural agency, psychogenic factors, or temporary remission? How one explains the phenomenon depends on one's explanatory framework.

Even more troubling than the extravagant claims made for faith healing by some religious salesmen and the inevitable disappointments that are sure to follow are the instances in which whole communities of faith reject medicine altogether. Believing that God intends Christians to seek healing exclusively by prayer and anointing, members of these communities permit no medical intervention and refuse all medical help for themselves and their families. Churches of this type are content to remain outside the public eye and to pursue their faith quietly. They find unwanted publicity from time to time when their members are prosecuted for the deaths of medically untreated members of their community, including their own children.[7]

Another branch of the faith-healing movement has been the gospel of health, wealth, and prosperity, which has been a highly visible emphasis of such independent evangelists as Kenneth Hagen (1917–2003) and Benny Hinn (b. 1952). By the use of carefully selected biblical texts, these evangelists have promised that all God's children—"Kingdom kids"—can expect God's material blessings in every area of life, including freedom from pain and sickness. Hagen maintained that it was always God's will that believers be healed of sickness and infirmity. The movement has enjoyed wide appeal both in prosperous Western countries and in countries that lack proper medical facilities and are characterized by endemic poverty.

Sectarian movements, including several that originated in America in the latter half of the nineteenth century, have not infrequently adopted alternative healing practices, which they incorporated as a distinctive element of their theology. In most cases these practices have focused on the encouragement of abstinence from addictive substances and the pursuit of a healthy lifestyle. Others have taken stands that have given them a reputation for opposing medicine. Jehovah's Witnesses, for example, in forbidding blood transfusions on the authority of novel interpretations of biblical texts, have caused tension among individual Witnesses who face the dilemma of whether to pursue a recommended medical procedure that might save a life or accept their church's opposition to that procedure.

A small minority of Christians have followed the second-century church father Origen in believing that truly spiritual Christians should rely on God for all healing, leaving those who are less spiritual to employ medicine. In every generation there have been some Christians who depended exclusively on religious healing for themselves. In many cases the decision has been an individual and sacrificial one, made at great personal cost. Christians have historically regarded suffering as a necessary element of living in this world that God sometimes uses for spiritual edification, but in most cases they have not actively sought it. One can raise few objections in cases where this path has been chosen in order to pursue a higher level of spirituality. Indeed, a singular life of faith that does not seek suffering but accepts it when it comes and desires the good to be gained from living with it may be commendable. It is one that was pursued by ascetics in the early church, and it has been pursued in modern times by believers who were willing to accept suffering joyfully in order to draw closer to God.

Less commendable is the practice of some ascetics to seek suffering for expiatory or purificatory ends by abusing or denying their bodies. These ascetics' mortification of the flesh sometimes manifested itself in extreme ways. The early hermit Macarius (fl. fourth century), as penance for having killed a fly in anger, permitted poisonous flies to sting his naked flesh for six months. Another, Simeon Stylites, sought to mortify the flesh by wrapping a rope tightly around his body until, after a year, the lacerated flesh produced an offensive stench. The abbot reprimanded him for his excessive mortification and asked him to leave the monastery. Such heroic mortification attracted those who saw it as a path to spiritual perfection, but more mature ascetics regarded it as extreme, believing that it entailed an excessive focus on the body that was spiritually harmful. The tradition, while not strong in our own day, will always be present in some branches of the monastic and ascetic tradition. It is based not on the denial of those elements that have been thought to deflect the soul from spiritual pursuits (the world, the flesh, and the devil) but rather on a dualistic view that regards the flesh (and the material world generally) as evil and only the spirit as good.

In every age, believers of certain religious traditions, among them Jews and Christians, have attributed some disease to demons. Where this belief has flourished, they have employed exorcism to cast out the malignant spirits who had allegedly caused the disease. Mental disease and epilepsy have often been popularly thought to be caused by demons because of the erratic behavior exhibited by those who were believed to be possessed. During the Babylonian captivity, some Jews assimilated the belief that disease could be attributed to demons and practiced exorcism in the Second Temple period. Modern writers in both the Protestant and Catholic traditions have produced a literature that testifies to their belief in demonic activity in such phenomena as the revival of interest in the occult in the 1970s. Less common has been the attribution of disease to demons, but it enjoys popularity especially among certain faith-healing groups who credit forms of mental illness and erratic behavior to demons. Sectarian healers have sometimes employed exorcism to treat disease that would normally result in institutionalization. When used in place of medical treatment, it tends to produce an unhealthy sensationalism and offers false hope for a situation in which institutional or professional care might have been more effective.

Not all those who have refused medicine and not all faith healers have opposed medicine. And while the attitudes toward medicine and physicians surveyed here have characterized several religious groups and faith communities, they have usually been found outside the central traditions of Christianity and indeed of all three Abrahamic faiths. They have usually been held by religious minorities, some, but not all, of which are termed marginal to mainstream religious groups. While those who maintained them believed that they were pursuing a divine purpose, they prevented their adherents from gaining treatment that could have assisted in their healing and perhaps saved their lives. Although they may have exhibited a deep personal faith by practicing self-denial, they have also produced unnecessary suffering, sometimes with tragic consequences. In these cases religion has been used with the best of intentions to hinder healing, not to assist it.

Suffering and Compassion

Few modern works of fiction have so deeply explored the human responses to apparently meaningless pain and suffering, without offering an explanation, as has Albert Camus's *The Plague* (1947).[8] A central figure is Father Paneloux, a Jesuit priest in the North African city of Oran, the site of a devastating plague. Father Paneloux is well read in the history of epidemic disease and in the literature of Christian theodicy. At the onset of the plague he delivers a sermon in which he presents a conventional approach. God sends plagues to call sinners to repentance, he says, and to lead those struck by the plague to the deeper spiritual life that is a consequence of their suffering. In a vivid picture of Christus Pantokrator (Christ the Judge), he tells his congregation that, failing repentance, "no earthly power, nay, not even—mark me well—the vaunted might of human science can avail you to avert the [divine] hand once it is stretched toward you. And winnowed, like corn on the bloodstained threshing floor of suffering, you will be cast away with the chaff."[9]

Father Paneloux seems to be speaking above, not to, his parishioners, and the tone of his sermon is judgmental and impersonal. Theodicies do not always comfort sufferers; indeed, they sometimes point them to judgment. Later, however, the priest becomes deeply touched by the distress caused by the plague. He has witnessed his parishioners' pain and the horror of an epidemic that invariably brings death to those it afflicts. In a second sermon, the triumphalism of conventional attempts to explain the disease has disappeared. His tone is no longer moralistic. He has been particularly touched by the affliction of the children around him. He identifies with their pain. He plunges into the wretched humanity of those who suffer. Within two weeks he contracts and dies of the plague.[10] It is through his participation in the pain of others that he acquires compassion for them.

The paradox of religious views of suffering, particularly those in the Jewish and Christian traditions, lies in the fact that the deepest feelings of compassion require suffering, not explanation, to sustain them. It is no accident that, in the virtue-based ethical systems that existed in classical society, compassion was not regarded as a virtue. In Greco-Roman culture, pity-based philanthropy was attributed to irrational motives. Similarly, in utilitarian ethics a rational approach finds little place for the discussion of the value of affliction. The goal is to reduce or eliminate it. In secular philosophical traditions a desire for the elimination of suffering has sometimes led to the demand that sufferers be put out of their misery. The philosophical justification for euthanasia has a long history that dates back to Plato. It is not found in the monotheistic traditions, whose adherents have sought to help the afflicted, not through healing alone, but by offering them spiritual solace that may not end their pain but does give it meaning. Distress elicits compassion, which does not call, as an attitude of mere kindness sometimes does, for the elimination of misery.

"Suffering," writes Laurie Zoloth, "presents [itself] as an interruption in being, a meaningless takeover of reason, and this rupture creates an opening, argues Emmanuel Levinas, that allow[s] a subject to respond, and in responding, create[s] the possibility of humanity, solidarity and loss in a tragic world. You have witnessed a loss, and you cannot hide, you must do whatever you can to restore the lost object, or in the case, a lost capacity, to the person in need."[11] Compassion is not a quality that grows instinctively in the human heart. Our natural inclinations work to crowd it out. It thrives best in the fertile soil of religious devotion, and it is touched by the suffering of humanity. Within the Jewish and Christian traditions it has been rooted in the love of God, which at its highest and deepest level fills the heart with a gratitude that overflows in active benevolence to those who bear the Creator's image. In all three of the Abrahamic faiths, compassion has historically been the root of a long history of medical beneficence. Beyond those faiths, compassion and kindness have often been expressed by physicians and other caregivers in communities where they have not been elevated to an ideal or grounded in a religious world-view. The ideal physician was a Greek creation. While the ethical ideal to extend charity in the practice of medicine was rare in classical society, it surely was extended by many physicians.

The modern spirit in medicine, whatever else may be credited to it, does not necessarily foster compassion. The best that medicine offers today grows out of the values that a nonreligious world-view encourages: medical positivism and the research that has provided us with our understanding of disease and its cure; and egalitarian health care, which strives to ensure that the finest medical attention is available to all without regard to gender or to social or economic distinction. I do not in the least deprecate these contributions to medical care when I say that an unintentional but perhaps inevitable result of the removal of religious values from health care has been to cut it off from the very source from which compassion springs.

Compassion is a quality that is fully compatible with scientific medicine and with progress in medical technology, but it is not one that grows naturally out of either. It is the desire to treat the sick person, not in a medically competent and professional manner alone, which was the Greek practice, but lovingly and tenderly as a human being who bears the image of God. It is an intentional and active virtue. Seeing our neighbors as worthy of care transforms medicine from a professional duty into a sacred calling, and the caregiver as one who willingly takes on the affliction of one's neighbor. As we do so, we become not merely outsiders who witness the pain of others but participants in their suffering. Compassionate care has no boundaries. It extends to all—in the parable of the Good Samaritan it includes one's ethnic and religious enemy—and it is not limited by the passage of time or to faith communities alone. Compassion is not a quality that can be called up at will. It can be desired, it can be encouraged, it can be cultivated. But without a transcendent and spiritual basis, it lacks the sustenance necessary to nurture and perfect it.

Notes

For each chapter an extensive bibliography of secondary literature on medicine and religion, with an emphasis on recent publications in English, is available at the publisher's website (www.press.jhu.edu); search for this book by title or by author for a link to the bibliography.

INTRODUCTION

1. George Washington suffered from a severe sore throat, for which he was bled three times in one day. First a pint of blood was removed; then, a few hours later, a second pint. In midafternoon his three physicians, after consultation, removed another quart of blood. On the evening of December 14, 1799, between ten and eleven o'clock, Washington passed away.

2. See on this point the remarks of Ludwig Edelstein in his review of William F. Petersen's *Hippocratic Wisdom: A Modern Appreciation of Ancient Scientific Achievement*, reprinted in *Ancient Medicine: Selected Papers of Ludwig Edelstein*, ed. Owsei Temkin and C. Lilian Temkin (Baltimore, 1967) 121–31.

3. See James Hannam, *Genesis of Science: How the Christian Middle Ages Launched the Scientific Revolution* (Washington, DC, 2011); and Ronald L. Numbers, ed., *Galileo Goes to Jail, and Other Myths about Science and Religion* (Cambridge, MA, 2009).

4. Darrel W. Amundsen, "Body, Soul, and Physician," in *Medicine, Society, and Faith in the Ancient and Medieval Worlds* (Baltimore, 1996) 2–5.

5. *The Shorter Oxford English Dictionary on Historical Principles*, 3rd ed., rev. with addenda by C. T. Onions (Oxford, 1972) 2:1697, s.v. "Religion."

6. Mary Lindeman, "Health and Disease," in *Encyclopedia of the Enlightenment*, ed. Alan Charles Kors (New York, 2003) 2:193.

7. Allan Young, "Health and Disease: Anthropological Perspectives," in *The Encyclopedia of Bioethics*, ed. Warren Thomas Reich, 2nd ed., rev. (New York, 1995) 2:1098–1100.

8. Blaise Pascal, *Pensées and the Provincial Letters*, trans. W. F. Trotter (New York, 1941) 95.

CHAPTER ONE: **The Ancient Near East**

1. According to Robert Biggs, "Sun-dried tablets have a certain durability if they don't get handled very much (contracts for land sales and such were often stored in pots where, if only taken out for examination in case of legal necessity, they tended to stay intact for years). Many of the tablets from the library of the Assyrian king Assurbanipal (r. 668–c. 627 BC) were baked [by fire], and these break and chip, but are as hard as bricks. Most

tablets were unbaked, and ordinarily when no longer useful would have been recycled to make new tablets. Many unbaked tablets in museums have simply disintegrated, largely due to humidity fluctuations, salt content, etc." Personal communication.

2. R. D. Biggs, "Medicine, Surgery, and Public Health in Ancient Mesopotamia," in *Civilizations of the Ancient Near East*, ed. J. M. Sasson (1995; reprint, Peabody, MA, 2000) 3:1913.

3. A. K. Shapiro and E. Shapiro claim that the fifteen remedies described on the oldest Sumerian medical tablet, which dates to c. 2100 BC, were placebos on the assumption that they had no healing properties. *The Powerful Placebo: From Ancient Priest to Modern Physician* (Baltimore, 1997) 3.

4. Trans. W. G. Lambert, quoted in Biggs, "Medicine, Surgery, and Public Health" 3:1918.

5. Hermann Hunger, *Spätbabylonische Texte aus Uruk* (Berlin, 1976), no. 46, lines 1–5, quoted in Biggs, "Medicine, Surgery, and Public Health" 3:1914.

6. According to tradition, which is overly schematic, Menes or Narmer united Upper and Lower Egypt. If they are names of historic pharaohs, they probably date to the pre-dynastic period.

7. K. R. Weeks, "Medicine, Surgery, and Public Health in Ancient Egypt," in Sasson, *Civilizations of the Ancient Near East* 3:1796. For the two papyri, see B. Ebbell, trans., *The Papyrus Ebers: The Greatest Egyptian Medical Document* (Copenhagen, 1937); and J. H. Breasted, ed., *The Edwin Smith Surgical Papyrus: Published in Facsimile and Hieroglyphic Transliteration, with Translation and Commentary*, 2 vols. (Chicago, 1930). A more recent translation of the latter can be found in J. P. Allen, *The Art of Medicine in Ancient Egypt* (New York, 2005) 72–115.

8. Breasted, *Edwin Smith Surgical Papyrus*, quoted in Weeks, "Medicine, Surgery, and Public Health" 3:1794.

9. Ibid., 3:1795, 1787.

10. Ibid., 3:1796; Allen, *Art of Medicine* 11.

11. Weeks, "Medicine, Surgery, and Public Health" 3:1789, 1787.

12. Ibid., 3:1791.

13. Ibid., 3:1789; Herodotus, *History* 2.37; Weeks, "Medicine, Surgery, and Public Health" 3:1793.

14. Weeks, "Medicine, Surgery, and Public Health" 3:1790.

15. Job 6:14; Ps. 35:13.

16. Gen. 1:26–27. See also Gen. 9:6 and Exod. 4:11.

17. Ps. 139:13–16; Jer. 1:5; Isa. 49:1. It has been maintained that the accidental destruction of the fetus in the controverted passage of Exodus 21:22–25 was not a capital offense but one that required monetary compensation. Walter Kaiser argues cogently, however, that the passage holds the death of an infant to be murder, which requires a life for a life. Walter C. Kaiser Jr., *Toward Old Testament Ethics* (Grand Rapids, MI, 1983) 168–72.

18. See Lev. 18:21, 20:2 (infanticide); and Exod. 1:17–21 and Ezek. 16:5 (exposure).

19. See, e.g., Ps. 51:16–17.

20. On the continuing problem of theodicy in Judaism, see N. Solomon, "From Folk Medicine to Bioethics in Judaism," in *Religion, Health and Suffering*, ed. John R. Hinnels and Roy Porter (London, 1999) 172–75.

21. Isa. 3:7; Ezek. 30:21; Isa. 1:6; Jer. 51:8, 8:22; Exod. 21:18–19.

22. Exod. 22:18; Lev. 19:26 and 31, 20:6 and 27; Deut. 18:10–11. For references to physicians, see Jer. 8:22; and 2 Chron. 16:12.

23. On divination, Exod. 22:18 and Deut. 18:10. On magic, Isa. 3:2–3; 2 Chron. 33:6; and Ezek. 13:18–20.

24. For examples of folk practices, see 2 Kings 20:7; Gen. 30:14–16; and 1 Kings 1:1–4.

25. The quotations are from Isa. 38:5, 21. See also 2 Kings 20, esp. v. 7.

26. See, e.g., Ps. 32:3–5, 38:1–11; Isa. 38:1–6; and 2 Sam. 12:16–23.

27. See J. Milgrom, *Leviticus 1–16: A New Translation with Introduction and Commentary*, Anchor Bible (New York, 1991) 718–36; and J. Klawans, "Concepts of Purity in the Bible," in *The Jewish Study Bible: Featuring the Jewish Publication Society Tanakh Translation*, ed. A. Berlin and Marc Z. Brettler (Oxford, 2004) 2041–47. These sources provide a convenient summary of Mary Douglas's influential views, for which see her *Purity and Danger: An Analysis of the Concepts of Pollution and Taboo* (New York, 1966) and *Leviticus as Literature* (Oxford, 1999).

28. See, e.g., Ps. 24:3–4; Job 33:9; Ps. 51:2, 10; and Klawans, "Concepts of Purity in the Bible" 2042.

29. W. F. Albright, *Yahweh and the Gods of Canaan* (Garden City, NY, 1968) 177–81. Albright's view has a long history, having been maintained by Maimonides, among others. For a critical evaluation, see Douglas, *Leviticus as Literature* 29–40.

30. Maimonides, *The Guide for the Perplexed* 3.48.

31. Klawans, "Concepts of Purity in the Bible" 2043.

32. Douglas, *Leviticus as Literature* 1–28. See also Klawans, "Concepts of Purity in the Bible" 2041, 2044.

33. Milgrom, *Leviticus 1–16* 725.

34. Lev. 13–14; Mk 1:40–42 [= Mt 8:2–3; Lk 5:12–14]; Lk 17:12. For the symptoms, see Lev. 13:1–44.

35. Sir. 30:14–17, esp. v. 16; 18:19; 37:30–31.

36. Sanhedrin 17B (surgeon); Shekalim 1–2 (temple physician). On compatibility, see S. T. Newmyer, "Talmudic Medicine and Greco-Roman Science: Crosscurrents and Resistance," in *Aufstieg und Niedergang der Römischen Welt* II.37, 3 (1996): 2904.

CHAPTER TWO: **Greece**

1. *Iliad* 1.9–52.

2. See, e.g., *Odyssey* 5.394–97.

3. Hesiod, *Works and Days*, trans. Glenn W. Most, Loeb Classical Library (Cambridge, MA, 2006), lines 90–92, 100–104, pp. 95–96.

4. A. W. H. Adkins, "Greek Religion," in *Historia Religionum: Handbook for the History of Religions*, ed. C. J. Bleeker and G. Widengren, vol. 1, *Religions of the Past* (Leiden, 1969) 404–5.

5. Plato, *Protagoras* 311b–c and *Phaedrus* 270c; Aristotle, *Politics* 1326a14; and Menon in *Anonymous Londinensis* 5–6.

6. "The Hippocratic Oath: Text, Translation and Interpretation," trans. Ludwig Edelstein, in *Ancient Medicine: Selected Papers of Ludwig Edelstein*, ed. Owsei Temkin and C. Lilian Temkin (Baltimore, 1967) 6.

7. Empedocles flourished c. 444–441 BC. The standard four humors are found in the Hippocratic treatise *On the Nature of Man*.

8. Herodotus, *History* 3.29–30.

9. For quotations from *The Sacred Disease*, see 1:139, 2:141, and 21:183. Translations of Hippocratic works are taken from the Loeb Classical Library edition of *Hippocrates*, vols. 1–4, trans. W. H. S. Jones and E. T. Withington (Cambridge, MA, 1923–31).

10. Epidemic diseases did not form an exception. Because they lacked clear visible external causes, such as blindness, skin disease, and sometimes even paralysis, they were grouped together with those types of disease that had a similar etiology.

11. Quotations are from *Regimen* 93.447 and 87.423 (*Hippocrates: Volume IV*, trans. W. H. S. Jones, Loeb Classical Library [Cambridge, MA, 1931]); and *Decorum*, 6.289 (*Hippocrates: Volume II*, trans. W. H. S. Jones, Loeb Classical Library [Cambridge, MA, 1923]).

12. Thucydides, *History of the Peloponnesian War*, trans. Rex Warner with an introduction and notes by M. I. Finley (London, 1974) 2.47–54.

13. Alexander D. Langmuir, Thomas D. Worthen, Jon Solomon, C. George Ray, and Eskild Peterson, "The Thucydides Syndrome," *New England Journal of Medicine* 313 (1985): 1027–30; D. M. Morens and M. C. Chu, "The Plague of Athens," ibid. 314 (1986): 855–56; A. J. Holladay, "The Thucydides Syndrome: Another View," ibid. 315 (1986): 1170–73; E. Baziotopoulou-Valavani, "A Mass Burial from the Cemetery of Kerameikos," in *Excavating Classical Culture: Recent Archaeological Discoveries in Greece* (Oxford, 2002) 187–201; M. Papagrigorakis, C. Yapijakis, S. Phillippos, and E. Baziotopoulou-Valavani, "DNA Examination of Ancient Dental Pulp Incriminates Typhoid Fever as Probable Cause of the Plague of Athens," *International Journal of Infectious Diseases* 10 (2006): 206–14. The proposed identification of typhoid fever has not been widely accepted.

14. Thucydides, *History* 2.51–53 (trans. Warner), pp. 154–55.

15. E. Edelstein and L. Edelstein, *Asclepius: A Collection and Interpretation of the Testimonies* (1945; reprint, Baltimore, 1998) 1:235, stele 2.30.

16. H. E. Sigerist, *History of Medicine* (London, 1961) 2:65–66.

17. Bronwen L. Wickkiser, *Asclepius, Medicine, and the Politics of Healing in Fifth-Century Greece: Between Craft and Cult* (Baltimore, 2008) 57 and n. 52.

18. Sophocles, *Ajax*, lines 581–82; Diodorus, frags. 30, 43.

CHAPTER THREE: **Rome**

1. *De agricultura* 141.

2. *Natural History* 29.5, 8. Translations of Pliny the Elder are taken from the Loeb Classical Library edition of the *Natural History*, trans. W. H. S. Jones (Cambridge, MA, 1963).

3. Plutarch, *Life of Cato* 23, translated by Ian Scott-Kilvert in *Makers of Rome: Nine Lives by Plutarch* (Baltimore, 1965).

4. Quoted in Pliny, *Natural History* 29.7.

5. Pliny, *Natural History* 30.1; Ulpian, *Digest* 50.13.1.3.

6. "Almost 90% of doctors in the 1st cent. AD, 75% in the 2nd, and 66% in the 3rd, are from the Greek East." Vivian Nutton, "Healers in the Medical Market Place: Towards a Social History of Graeco-Roman Medicine," in *Medicine in Society: Historical Essays*, ed. A. Wear (Cambridge, 1992) 39.

7. G. E. R. Lloyd, *Demystifying Mentalities* (Cambridge, 1990) 30–31; Vivian Nutton,

"Murders and Miracles: Lay Attitudes towards Medicine in Classical Antiquity," reprinted in *From Democedes to Harvey: Studies in the History of Medicine* (London, 1988) VIII 40.

8. Vivan Nutton, "Roman Medicine: Tradition, Confrontation, Assimilation," *Aufstieg und Niedergang der Römischen Welt* II.37, 1 (1993): 76 and n. 116.

9. Nutton, "Healers in the Medical Market Place" 38–49.

10. All 732 are listed and described by Jürgen W. Riethmüller in *Asklepios: Heiligtümer und Kulte*, 2 vols. (Heidelberg, 2005).

11. See A. D. Nock, *Conversion: The Old and the New in Religion from Alexander the Great to Augustine of Hippo* (1933; reprint, London, 1961) 83–93.

12. E. R. Dodds, *Pagan and Christian in an Age of Anxiety: Some Aspects of Religious Experience from Marcus Aurelius to Constantine* (Cambridge, 1968) 39–45, quotation from 42. For Dodds's retrospective psychoanalysis, see 41–43. See also André-Jean Festugière, *Personal Religion among the Greeks* (Berkeley and Los Angeles, 1960) 85–104. Marcus Aurelius's adoptive father, Antoninus Pius (r. 138–61) was, before he ascended the throne, already a supporter of Asclepius's cult and had constructed new buildings at his shrine in Epidaurus.

13. Elizabeth Ann Leeper, "Exorcism in Early Christianity" (PhD diss., Duke University, 1991) 177–79; Peter Brown, *The World of Late Antiquity* (New York, 1972) 49–57; Nock, *Conversion* 104–5.

14. Against this view, see Gary B. Fengren, *Medicine and Health Care in Early Christianity* (Baltimore, 2009) 54–57.

15. *Enneads* 2.9.14. The passage is quoted and translated by Ludwig Edelstein in *Ancient Medicine: Selected Papers of Ludwig Edelstein*, ed. Owsei Temkin and C. Lilian Temkin (Baltimore, 1967) 221. On Gnosticism, see J. Doresse, "Gnosticism," in *Historia Religionum: Handbook for the History of Religions*, ed. C. J. Bleeker and G. Widengren, vol. 1, *Religions of the Past* (Leiden, 1969) 533–79.

16. On Jewish amulets in the ancient and medieval periods, see L. H. Schiffman and M. D. Swartz, *Hebrew and Aramaic Incantation Texts from the Cairo Genizah: Selected Texts from Taylor-Schechter Box K1* (Sheffield, UK, 1992) 11–62. The Cairo Genizah texts date from the medieval period. On Eleazar, see Josephus, *Antiquities* 8.2.5. Often cited in support of Solomon's incantations were 1 Kings 5:12 and Wisd. of Sol. 7:15–22.

CHAPTER FOUR· **Early Christianity**

1. See, e.g., Mt 11:4–5, which echoes Isa. 35:4–6 and 61:1 (fulfilled prophecy); Jn 1:37 38 (miracles as signs); Mt 8:16, with which cf. Mk 6:12 and Acts 19:12 (exorcism and healing).

2. Mt 25:35–36, 45. The verb *epeskepsasthe* (from *episkopein*), used in this passage to mean taking care of the sick, is sometimes employed in late classical Greek to describe a physician's visiting a patient.

3. Lk 10:25–37.

4. Darrel Amundsen tells me, however, that it was not so used in the early church.

5. James 5:14–16 (prayer and anointing), 5:10–11 (Job).

6. *Contra Celsum* 3.12.

7. On maturity, see, e.g., Heb. 12:7–11 and 1 Pet. 4:12. On Christian graces, see Rom. 5:2–5; James 5:10–11; and 2 Cor. 12:7–10.

8. Thucydides, *History* 2.52; Eusebius, *Ecclesiastical History* 7:22.

9. See Mk 9:38–40; Lk 9:49–50; and Acts 19:13–16.

10. Mt 9:32–33, Lk 11:14; Mt 12:22; Mt 17:14–20, Mk 9:14–29, Lk 9:37–43.

11. See, e.g., Mk 5:1–5 and Mt 8:28–29 (erratic behavior); the case of the paralytic in Jn 5:2–9 (healing); and Mk 5:24–34 (chronic illness).

12. Peter Brown, *Augustine of Hippo: A Biography* (1969; reprint, Berkeley and Los Angeles, 2000) 419.

13. Peter Brown, "The Rise and Function of the Holy Man In Late Antiquity," *Journal of Roman Studies* 61 (1971) 99.

14. See Peregrine Horden, "The Death of Ascetics: Sickness and Monasticism in the Early Byzantine Middle East," reprinted in his *Hospitals and Healing from Antiquity to the Later Middle Ages* (Aldershot, UK, 2008), essay X, 41–52.

15. Rowan A. Greer, *The Fear of Freedom: A Study of Miracles in the Roman Imperial Church* (University Park, PA, 1989) 180–81.

16. Eusebius, *Ecclesiastical History* 6.43.

17. Adolf Harnack, *The Mission and Expansion of Christianity in the First Three Centuries*, trans. and ed. James Moffat, 3 vols. (New York, 1904) 1:195n1; John Chrysostrom, *Homily on Matthew* 66/67.3.

18. *New History* 1.26, 37; see also 1.36, 46.

19. Rodney Stark, *The Rise of Christianity: A Sociologist Reconsiders History* (Princeton, NJ, 1996) 206, emphasis original.

20. Quoted in Eusebius, *Ecclesiastical History* 7.22.7.

21. *Apology* 40.

22. Cyprian, *Ad Demetrianum* 2, 10–11; Pontius, *Vita Cypriani* 9–11.

23. Gregory of Nyssa, *Vita Gregorii Thaumaturgi* 12; for Dionysius, see Eusebius, *Ecclesiastical History* 7.22.

24. Tertullian, *Apology* 39.6; Aristides, *Apology* 15 (burial); Julian, *Epistle to Arsacius* 49.

25. Stark, *Rise of Christianity* 74–75, 89, emphasis original. See the discussion of differential mortality on pp. 88–91.

26. Andrew Todd Crislip, *From Monastery to Hospital: Christian Monasticism and the Transformation of Health Care in Late Antiquity* (Ann Arbor, MI, 2005) 101–2.

27. Gregory of Nazianzus, *Oration* 20.

28. Jerome, *Epistle* 77 (Fabiola). Julian, *Epistle to Arsacius* 49; cf. 22.

CHAPTER FIVE: **The Middle Ages**

1. A first-century description of the Germans written by a distinguished Roman historian can be found in Tacitus's *Germania*. Their tribal names do not necessarily represent specific different ethnic identities but are labels invented by the Romans and modern historians. See Patrick J. Geary, *The Myth of Nations: The Medieval Origins of Europe* (Princeton, NJ, 2002).

2. For a popular treatment of this view, see Peter S. Wells, *Barbarians to Angels: The Dark Ages Reconsidered* (New York, 2008).

3. F. C. Finucane, *Miracles and Pilgrims: Popular Beliefs in Medieval England* (1977; reprint, New York, 1995) 10–11.

4. This was the practice of accommodation, which allowed Christian converts to re-

tain some seemingly harmless pagan institutions in order to make the transition to the new faith easier. On the characteristic features of Germanic religion, see H. R. Ellis Davidson, "Germanic Religion," in *Historia Religionum: Handbook for the History of Religions*, ed. C. J. Bleeker and G. Widengren, vol. 1, *Religions of the Past* (Leiden, 1969) 611–28.

5. Most monastic infirmaries did not become separate hospitals until the eleventh century.

6. J. Kroll, "Mental Health and Illness," in *Encyclopedia of the Middle Ages*, ed. Norman F. Cantor (New York, 1999) 1124.

7. D. W. Amundsen, "The Medieval Catholic Tradition," in *Caring and Curing: Health and Medicine in the Western Religious Traditions*, ed. Ronald L. Numbers and Darrel W. Amundsen (1986; reprint, Baltimore, 1997) 75–76.

8. N. G. Siraisi, *Medieval and Early Renaissance Medicine: An Introduction to Knowledge and Practice* (Chicago, 1990) 10–11. For an example of the mingling of medicine and religious healing, as well as the Christian aversion to charms and spells, see the example of Francesca Romana, who cared for the sick poor, on pp. 44–46.

9. Rule 1.31; Cassiodorus, *Introduction to Divine and Human Readings*, trans. Leslie Webber Jones (New York, 1946).

10. *De vitis partum Emeritensium* 4.

11. See L. C. MacKinney, "Medical Ethics and Etiquette in the Early Middle Ages: The Persistence of Hippocratic Ideals," *Bulletin of the History of Medicine* 26 (1952): 1–31; and Darrel Amundsen and Gary Ferngren, "Medicine and Religion: Early Christianity through the Middle Ages," in *Health/Medicine and the Faith Traditions: An Inquiry into Religion and Medicine*, ed. Martin E. Marty and Kenneth L. Vaux (Philadelphia, 1982) 119–20.

12. See M. Green, ed. and trans., *The "Trotula": A Medieval Compendium of Women's Medicine* (Philadelphia, 2001) 3–14.

13. Siraisi, *Medieval and Early Renaissance Medicine* 86–89. Despite frequent statements to the contrary, the church never forbade human dissection in medical schools. For the reasons that prevented its being practiced, see ibid., 88–91.

14. Jerome Bylebyl "distinguished between the empirically-trained *medicus* (doctor) and the *physicus* (physician), who had received university medical training. The university-trained physician was relatively rare, compared to the wide range of other kinds of doctors, surgeons, empirical healers, et al." The latter were trained by apprenticeship. Harry York, in a personal communication.

15. John Riddle wrote in a personal communication, "I have seldom seen in medical documents indications that astrology was a regular part of practice. To be sure, there are theoretical works that assert this but I can't find a link with practice (except the one find of a vade mecum)."

16. M. McVaugh, *Medicine before the Plague: Practitioners and their Patients in the Crown of Aragon, 1285–1345* (Cambridge, 1993) 140–41.

17. Siraisi, *Medieval and Early Renaissance Medicine* 27.

18. Amundsen and Ferngren, "Medicine and Religion" 117.

19. The hospital has served a variety of functions since its founding. See Guenter B. Risse, in *Mending Bodies, Saving Souls: A History of Hospitals* (New York, 1999); and Mary Lindemann, *Medicine and Society in Early Modern Europe* (Cambridge, 2010) 159.

20. *Psychosomatic medicine* is Peregrine Horden's term. See Ferngren, *Medicine and Health Care* 130.

21. L. I. Conrad, *The Western Medical Tradition: 800 BC to AD 1800* (Cambridge, 1995) 71–87, 150–52.

22. On the nature and definitions of leprosy in the Middle Ages and earlier, see L. E. Demaitre, *Leprosy in Premodern Medicine: A Malady of the Whole Body* (Baltimore, 2007) 80–131; on the incidence of the disease, see Cartwright, *Social History of Medicine* 58.

23. In 2011 a research team at McMaster University discovered the now-extinct variant of the *Yersinia pestis* bacterium that caused the Black Death. They analyzed the DNA from the teeth of four human skeletons taken from the site of a mass grave in London that dated from 1349. "Plague bug wasn't all that fierce," *Science News* 108, no. 11 (November 19, 2011): 18. The Black Death cannot be identified with the bubonic plague of modern times, and some historians have attacked the conventional reconstruction of the disease and how it was spread. See V. Nutton, ed., *Pestilential Complexities: Understanding Medieval Plague* (London, 2008).

24. Siraisi, *Medieval and Early Renaissance Medicine* 18–29.

25. Motives were undoubtedly mixed. Chaucer states that his own physician remained to treat those afflicted with the plague. He did it, says Chaucer, not out of charity but to charge high fees for his treatment.

26. Elisabeth Carniel, "Plague Today," in Nutton, *Pestilential Complexities* 115.

27. K. Park, "Medicine and Society in Medieval Europe, 500–1500," in *Medicine in Society: Historical Essays*, ed. A. Wear (Cambridge, 1992) 73.

28. Finucane, *Miracles and Pilgrims* 67. See also J. Duffin, *Medical Miracles: Doctors, Saints, and Healing in the Modern World* (Oxford, 2009) 72; and Park, "Medicine and Society" 72.

29. The tension between those favoring *theoria* and those favoring *praxis* led to disputes between bishops and urban monks over what constituted the proper monastic life and whether monks should serve in hospitals. T. Miller, *The Birth of the Hospital in the Byzantine Empire* (Baltimore, 1997) 118–22.

30. P. Horden, "How Medicalised Were Byzantine Hospitals?," *Medicina e Storia* 5 (2006): 49–50.

31. See E. Wipszycka, "Les confréries dans la vie religieuse de l'Egypte chretienne," in *Proceedings of the Twelfth International Congress of Papyrology*, ed. D. H. Samuel, American Studies in Papyrology 7 (Toronto, 1970) 513–15; and P. Horden, "The Confraternities of Byzantium," in *Voluntary Religion*, ed. W. P. Sheils and Diana Wood (Oxford, 1986) 40.

32. For a representative collection of the attested miracles of Saint John Prodromouos, see *The Miracles of St. Artemios: A Collection of Miracle Stories by an Anonymous Author of Seventh-Century Byzantium*, trans. Virgil S. Crisafulli with an introduction by John W. Nesbitt (Leiden, 1996). Miracle 22 provides an interesting account of the cooperation of physicians in a hospital with the supernatural healing of Saint Artemios.

33. John Scarborough, "The Life and Times of Alexander of Tralles," *Expedition* 39, no. 2 (1997): 55.

CHAPTER SIX: **Islam in the Middle Ages**

1. I. Ilkilic, "The Discourses of Islamic Medical Ethics," in *The Cambridge World History of Medical Ethics*, ed. Robert B. Baker and Laurence B. McCullough (New York, 2009) 270.

2. The common historical narrative traces the origins of the Shia and Sunni branches of Islam to the succession dispute after the death of the Prophet. However, many historians do not believe that there is enough historical evidence to trace the development of Shiite theology or politics in the eighth and ninth centuries to that early event, which they maintain is largely a teleological and anachronistic reading.

3. Ilkilic, "Discourses of Islamic Medical Ethics" 271, 276.

4. F. *Rahman, "Islam and Health/Medicine: A Historical Perspective," in Healing and Restoring: Health and Medicine in the World's Religious Traditions*, ed. L. E. Sullivan (New York, 1989) 177; Ilkilic, "Discourses of Islamic Medical Ethics" 270–71.

5. Rahman, "Islam and Health/Medicine" 157; I. Ilkilic, "Medical Ethics through the Life Cycle in the Islamic Middle East," in Baker and McCullough, *Cambridge World History of Medical Ethics* 168; Quran 67:2, 21:35, 38:41–44, 17:23. All quotations from the Quran are from Muhammad Asad's translation.

6. M. Dols, *Majnūn: The Madman in Medieval Islamic Society* (Oxford, 1992) 245–46.

7. Quran 17:82, 26:78–80.

8. Dols, *Majnūn* 244; Rahman, "Islam and Health/Medicine" 155; Ilkilic, "Discourses of Islamic Medical Ethics" 271, 168–69; Rahman, "Islam and Health/Medicine" 156; Dols, *Majnūn* 227.

9. Rahman, "Islam and Health/Medicine" 151; L. I. Conrad, "Arab-Islamic Medicine," in *Companion Encyclopedia of the History of Medicine*, ed. W. F. Bynum and R. Porter (London, 1993) 1:678–79, 683.

10. Rahman, "Islam and Health/Medicine" 151; S. H. Nasr, *Islamic Science: An Illustrated Study* (London, 1976) 174–76.

11. U. Weisser, "The Discourse of Practitioners in the Ninth to Fourteenth Century Middle East," in Baker and McCullough, *Cambridge World History of Medical Ethics* 363; Nasr, *Islamic Science* 154; Quran 67:2–3; P. E. Pormann and E. Savage-Smith, *Medieval Islamic Medicine* (Edinburgh, 2007) 32–33.

12. Conrad, "Arab-Islamic Medicine" 1:697–98.

13. Muslim physicians are also known for some medical practices and innovations vis-à-vis Greek medicine. Examples are ophthalmology and the removal of cataracts, as well as surgical procedures, such as removing kidney and bladder stones.

14. Ilkilic, "Discourses of Islamic Medical Ethics" 273; Weisser, "Discourse of Practitioners" 368.

15. Nasr, *Islamic Science* 154, 163; Quran 51:20–21.

16. Pormann and Savage-Smith, *Medieval Islamic Medicine* 136; Nasr, *Islamic Science* 157.

17. Quran 11:20, 3:92, 2:261; Rahman, "Islam and Health/Medicine" 153.

18. Pormann and Savage-Smith, *Medieval Islamic Medicine* 97, 100 (quotation).

19. Ibid., 101–2; Weisser, "Discourse of Practitioners" 364; Rahman, "Islam and Health/Medicine" 152–53, 159.

20. Weisser, "Discourse of Practitioners" 367–68; S. H. Nasr, *Science and Civilization in Islam* (Cambridge, 1987) 184–85.

21. Ilkilic, "Discourses of Islamic Medical Ethics" 276; Weisser, "Discourse of Practitioners" 367.

22. Nasr, *Islamic Science* 166.

23. It was, however, permissible to use alcohol externally.

24. Dols, *Majnūn* 243–52.

25. Pormann and Savage-Smith, *Medieval Islamic Medicine* 71–73; Ilkilic, "Discourses of Islamic Medical Ethics" 272–73; Conrad, "Arab-Islamic Medicine" 1:707–8.

26. Dols, *Majnūn* 211, 233–35.

27. To this day pilgrims take back to the holy centers of their Islamic lands the water of Zamzam, a well located in Makkah, to be used not only for blessing but also for healing.

28. Rahman, "Islam and Health/Medicine" 151; Nasr, *Islamic Science* 172; Pormann and Savage-Smith, *Medieval Islamic Medicine* 145.

CHAPTER SEVEN: **The Early Modern Period**

1. E. Harris Harbison, "The Protestant Reformation," in *Christianity and History* (Princeton, NJ, 1964) 141–56. On the unexpected long-term results of the Reformation, see Brad S. Gregory, *The Unintended Reformation: How a Religious Revolution Secularized Society* (Cambridge, MA, 2012).

2. J. M. Gustafson, *Protestant and Roman Catholic Ethics: Prospects for Rapprochement* (Chicago, 1978) 3–6; Harbison, "Protestant Reformation" 148–50.

3. E. L. Eisenstein, *The Printing Press as an Agent of Change: Communications and Cultural Transformations in Early-Modern Europe* (Cambridge, 1979) 2:636–82. Eisenstein suggests that finding a printer was a greater determining factor than was the Index for the dissemination of ideas and that natural philosophers created correspondence networks of dissemination that transcended national boundaries and religious differences (2:642–43).

4. For the early Protestant view of the cessation of miracles, see Keith Thomas, *Religion and the Decline of Magic* (New York, 1971) 124–25; B. B. Warfield, *Counterfeit Miracles* (1918; reprint, London, 1972) 306n25; and Colin Brown, *Miracles and the Critical Mind* (Grand Rapids, MI, 1984) 13–18.

5. J. Sidlow Baxter, *Divine Healing of the Body* (Grand Rapids, MI, 1979) 77–89. On John Wesley, see Deborah Madden, *A Cheap, Safe and Natural Medicine: Religion, Medicine and Culture in John Wesley's Primitive Physic* (Amsterdam, 2007).

6. For a survey of this much-discussed question, see E. B. Davis and M. P. Winship, "Early-Modern Protestantism," in *The History of Science and Religion in the Western Tradition: An Encyclopedia*, ed. G. B. Ferngren (New York, 2000) 281–87.

7. C. Lindberg, "The Lutheran Tradition," in *Caring and Curing: Health and Medicine in the Western Religious Traditions*, ed. Ronald L. Numbers and Darrel W. Amundsen (1986; reprint, Baltimore, 1997), quotations from 178; J. H. Smylie, "The Reformed Tradition," in ibid., 208–12.

8. R. L. Numbers and R. C. Sawyer, "Medicine and Christianity in the Modern World," in *Health/Medicine and the Faith Traditions: An Enquiry into Religion and Medicine*, ed. Martin E. Marty and Kenneth L. Vaux (Philadelphia, 1982) 138 and nn. 9–11. Paré was reputed to have been either a Huguenot or sympathetic to the Huguenot cause and to have narrowly escaped death during the St. Bartholomew's Day Massacre, but he remained a Catholic all his life. On the alleged Huguenot sympathies of Paré, see J. F. Malgaigne, *Surgery and Ambrose Paré*, trans. and ed. Wallace B. Hamby, MD (Norman, OK, 1965) 287–92. His dictum reflects broadly Christian rather than sectarian assumptions.

On Carlstadt, see Warfield, *Counterfeit Miracles* 306n26. On Edinburgh, see Guenter B. Risse, *Mending Bodies, Saving Souls: A History of Hospitals* (New York, 1999) 237–38.

9. See Sachiko Kusukawa, *The Transformation of Natural Philosophy: The Case of Philip Melanchthon* (Cambridge, 1995).

10. Vesalius was not the first to perform dissections himself. He was inspired to do so by a Latin translation of Galen. Nor did he reject texts altogether; as a humanist he wanted better texts. On the Wittenberg anatomy, see Roger French, *Medicine before Science: The Rational and Learned Doctor from the Middle Ages to the Enlightenment* (Cambridge, 2003) 147–48.

11. A. Wear, "The Popularization of Medicine in Early Modern England," in *The Popularization of Medicine, 1650–1850*, ed. R. Porter (London, 1992) 288–89. On natural history, see French, *Medicine before Science* 150–51.

12. On Paracelsus, see Walter Pagel, *Paracelsus* (Basel, 1958). For a treatment of Paracelsus's heterodox Christianity, see Charles Webster, *Paracelsus: Medicine, Magic, and Mission at the End of Time* (New Haven, CT, 2008). On his apocalypticism, see Wear, "Popularization of Medicine" 312. On empiricism in Protestantism, see Davis and Winship, "Early-Modern Protestantism" 282.

13. On the interpretation of astrology, see W. R. Newman and L. M. Principe, "Some Problems with the Historiography of Alchemy," in *Secrets of Nature: Astrology and Alchemy in Early Modern Europe*, ed. W. R. Newman and A. Grafton (2001; reprint, Cambridge, MA, 2006 [2001]) 385–431.

14. Wear, "Popularization of Medicine" 323, 298–99.

15. For one example of popular healing, the *pauliani*, see Katharine Park, "Country Medicine in the City Marketplace: Snakehandlers as Itinerant Healers," *Renaissance Studies* 15 (2001): 104–20; on traveling medical charlatans, see M. A. Katritzky, "Marketing Medicine: The Image of the Early Modern Mountebank," ibid., 121–53; on the popularity of amulets and jewelry, see John Cherry, "Healing through Faith: The Continuation of Medieval Attitudes to Jewellery in the Renaissance," ibid., 154–71.

16. R. Porter, introduction to Porter, *Popularization of Medicine* 1–2, 30–33.

17. Natalie Zemon Davis argued that religious factors did not influence the transformation of poor relief in the sixteenth and seventeenth centuries, which she said resulted chiefly from recent economic and demographic changes. "Poor Relief, Humanism and Heresy," in *Society and Culture in Early Modern France* (Stanford, 1975) 17–64. More recent scholarship has emphasized, however, that medical-relief reforms in the sixteenth and seventeenth centuries were largely the result of ideological and political factors, especially those of the Protestant Reformation. See Ole Peter Grell and Andrew Cunningham, "The Reformation and Changes in Welfare Provision in Early Modern Northern Europe," in *Health Care and Poor Relief in Protestant Europe, 1500–1700*, ed. Grell and Cunningham (London, 1997) 1–42, esp. 2 and the literature cited in 32n2. While the economic and social changes should not be underestimated, Grell has demonstrated that Protestant and Christian humanist ideas provided the motivation for the rapid changes that occurred. Ole Peter Grell, "The Protestant Imperative of Christian Care and Neighbourly Love," in ibid., 43–65.

18. Grell and Cunningham, "Reformation and Changes in Welfare Provision" 3–4; Grell, "Protestant Imperative" 49–52; C. Lindberg, "The Liturgy after the Liturgy: Wel-

fare in the Early Reformation," in *Through the Eye of the Needle: Judeo-Christian Roots of Social Welfare*, ed. E. Hanawalt and C. Lindberg (Kirksville, MO, 1994) 177–91.

19. Grell, "Protestant Imperative" 58; T. Riis, "Religion and Early Modern Social Welfare," in Hanawalt and Lindberg, *Through the Eye of the Needle* 193–205; Grell and Cunningham, "Reformation and Changes in Welfare Provision" 28; Grell, "Protestant Imperative" 53–57.

20. Michel Foucault (1926–1984) argued that the creation of institutions for the insane, criminals, and the poor in the mid-seventeenth century constituted a "great confinement" that sought to incarcerate deviants in order to discipline them and teach them to work. See his *Madness and Civilization: A History of Insanity in the Age of Reason* (New York, 1973) and *Discipline and Punish: The Birth of the Prison* (1977; reprint, New York, 1995). For a critique of Foucault's views regarding "the manufacture of madness," see C. Jones and R. Porter, eds., *Reassessing Foucault: Power, Medicine, and the Body* (London, 1994); and Grell, "Protestant Imperative" 60.

21. A. Kinzelbach, "Hospitals, Medicine, and Society: Southern German Imperial Towns in the Sixteenth Century," *Renaissance Studies* 15 (2001): 217–28, esp. 219–21.

22. E. I. Kouri, "Health Care and Poor Relief in Sweden and Finland: c. 1500–1700," in Grell and Cunningham, *Health Care and Poor Relief* 179–80; Grell and Cunningham, "Reformation and Changes in Welfare Provision" 23–33, quotation from 32–33.

23. John Henderson, "Healing the Body and Saving the Soul: Hospitals in Renaissance Florence," *Renaissance Studies* 15 (2001): 216. For more on hospitals and poor relief in southern Italy, see ibid., 188–216; and D. Gentilcore, *Healers and Healing in Early Modern Europe* (Manchester, UK, 1998) 125–55. On Flanders, see Hugo Soly, "Continuity and Change: Attitudes towards Poor Relief and Health Care in Early Modern Antwerp," in Grell and Cunningham, *Health Care and Poor Relief* 90.

24. See Brian S. Pullan, *Rich and Poor in Renaissance Venice: The Social Institutions of a Catholic State, 1650* (Oxford, 1971); Grell and Cunningham, "Reformation and Changes in Welfare Provision" 19; and Wear, "Popularization of Medicine" 244–50.

25. Porter, *Popularization of Medicine* 102–3.

26. Ibid.

27. See L. Pollock, *With Faith and Physic: The Life of a Tudor Gentlewoman, Lady Grace Mildmay, 1552–1620* (New York, 1995), esp. 92–109 and 110–42, quotation from 92. On her religious life, see 48–69 and 70–91.

28. On Protestant asceticism, which was adopted by John Wesley and became a part of his "method," see Anita Guerrini, *Obesity and Depression in the Enlightenment: The Life and Times of George Cheyne* (Norman, OK, 2000) 139–52.

29. P. Kocher, "The Idea of God in Elizabethan Medicine," *Journal of the History of Ideas* 11 (1950): 6–7.

30. Cotton Mather, *The Angel of Bethesda: An Essay upon the Common Maladies of Mankind*, ed. G. W. Jones (Barre, MA, 1972).

31. Harbison, "Protestant Reformation" 152–55.

32. Gustafson, *Protestant and Roman Catholic Ethics* 3, 132; Allen Verhey, "Protestantism," in *The Encyclopedia of Bioethics*, ed. Warren T. Reich, 2nd ed., rev. (New York, 1995) 4:2117–18, 2123–24; Harbison, "Protestant Reformation" 145.

33. On Baxter, see Smylie, "Reformed Tradition" 212.

34. Charles Webster, *The Great Instauration: Science, Medicine, and Reform, 1626–1660* (London, 1975). On Bacon's influence on Boyle and the Royal Society, see Rose-May Sargent, *The Diffident Naturalist* (Chicago, 1995). Webster and Peter Harrison (*The Fall of Man and the Foundations of Science* [Cambridge, 2007]) both discuss Bacon's notion of the prolongation of life, a subject that would prove to be very influential throughout the seventeenth and eighteenth centuries. On common-sense philosophy, see Walter H. Conser, "Baconianism," in Ferngren, *History of Science and Religion* 169–71.

35. A. R. Jonsen, *A Short History of Medical Ethics* (New York, 2000) 57–67.

36. P. A. Watson, *The Angelical Conjunction: The Preacher-Physicians of Colonial New England* (Knoxville, TN, 1991); Wear, "Popularization of Medicine" 240; Numbers and Sawyer, "Medicine and Christianity" 140.

37. Mather, "The Angel of Bethesda," quoted in Smylie, "Reformed Tradition" 213.

38. On Mather, see Smylie, "Reformed Tradition" 212–13; and Mary Lindemann, *Medicine and Society in Early Modern Europe* (Cambridge, 2010) 76–77, with citations to recent literature. On Wesley and the early Methodist movement, see Guerrini, *Obesity and Depression in the Enlightenment* 184; and H. D. Rack, "Doctors, Demons, and Early Methodist Healing," in *The Church and Healing*, ed. W. J. Sheils (Oxford, 1982) 137–52, which exaggerates the "irrationality" and "religious hysteria" of Wesley and his followers.

39. Numbers and Sawyer, "Medicine and Christianity" 136; J. Duffy, "Anglo-American Reaction to Obstetrical Anesthesia," *Bulletin of the History of Medicine* 38 (1964): 32–44; C. A. Russell, "Objections to Anaesthesia: The Case of James Young Simpson," in *Gases in Medicine: Anaesthesia*, ed. E. B. Smith and S. Daniels (Cambridge, 1998).

40. See G. Ferngren, "The Ethics of Suicide in the Renaissance and Reformation," in *Suicide and Euthanasia: Historical and Contemporary Themes*, ed. B. A. Brody (Dordrecht, 1989) 155–81.

41. Quoted in K. L. Sprunger, *The Learned Doctor William Ames: Dutch Backgrounds of English and American Puritanism* (Urbana, IL, 1972) 153.

42. M. R. O'Connell, "The Roman Catholic Tradition Since 1545," in Numbers and Amundsen, *Caring and Curing* 115.

43. See Gentilcore, *Healers and Healing* 156–73. Gentilecore points out that the chief function of saints was to perform miracle cures (178). Living saints were often women. On the survival of Catholic pilgrimage, see J. Sumption, *Pilgrimage: An Image of Medieval Religion* (Totowa, NJ, 1975) 300–302. On canonization, see J. Duffin, *Medical Miracles: Doctors, Saints, and Healing in the Modern World* (Oxford, 2009). Duffin describes specific diseases reportedly healed by candidates for sainthood (73–111) and provides comparative tables of diseases cured from the sixteenth to the twentieth centuries.

44. O'Connell, "Roman Catholic Tradition Since 1545" 120, 128.

45. Numbers and Sawyer, "Medicine and Christianity" 143–44.

46. M. Lindemann, "Health and Disease," in *Encyclopedia of the Enlightenment*, ed. Alan Charles Kors (New York, 2003) 2:193.

47. Numbers and Sawyer, "Medicine and Christianity" 146; G. B. Risse, "Hospitals," in Kors, *Encyclopedia of the Enlightenment* 2:220.

48. Quoted in Porter, *Popularization of Medicine* 384. See also Lindemann, "Health and Disease" 2:194. Descartes himself relied heavily on physiology, to which he devoted much time (including dissection), in creating what was a materialist philosophical sys-

tem. H. J. Cook, "Medicine," in *The Cambridge History of Science*, vol. 3, *Early Modern Science*, ed. K. Park and L. Daston (New York, 2006) 427–29. On the debate over whether the Enlightenment produced much real medical progress, see Porter, *Popularization of Medicine* 380–81, citing the opinions of Fielding Garrison and Peter Gay.

49. Lindemann, "Health and Disease" 2:194; Numbers and Sawyer, "Medicine and Christianity" 142–43.

50. For a summary treatment of the variety of healers who practiced medicine in early modern Europe, see Lindemann, *Medicine and Society* 235–80; and Maria Bogucka, "Health Care and Poor Relief in Danzig (Gdansk)," in Grell and Cunningham, *Health Care and Poor Relief* 214–15. Barber-surgeons treated broken bones, hernias, cataracts, and other diseases of the body's exterior.

51. Lindemann, *Medicine and Society* 156, 258.

52. The terms *mountebank* and *quacksalver* (from which *quack*) were commonly used for medical imposters.

53. Porter, *Popularization of Medicine* 413–14.

54. Lindemann, *Medicine and Society* 272–77.

55. F. F. Cartwright, *A Social History of Medicine* (London, 1977) 134–35.

CHAPTER EIGHT: **The Nineteenth and Twentieth Centuries**

1. Scholarly disagreement exists regarding whether the First Great Awakening was a historical event or rather an "interpretive fiction" created by historians. Jon Butler, *Awash in a Sea of Faith: Christianizing the American People* (Cambridge, MA, 1990), argues that the First Great Awakening was a series of isolated, regionally specific revivals that occurred within Protestant congregations. Against this view, Thomas S. Kidd, *The Great Awakening: A Brief History with Documents* (Boston, 2008), maintains that the revivals had a lasting influence beyond their limited effect on levels of religiosity in the American colonies.

2. While concern for evangelism was one of the reasons evangelicals pursued social reform in the nineteenth century, their activities in the United States were firmly grounded in theological tendencies toward perfectionism (and eventually holiness) and postmillennialism that emerged in the Second Great Awakening. Social reform grew from increasing evangelical assent to ideas that all humans could be saved, that God's revelation was ongoing and direct, that twice-born people could be perfected, and that through individual redemption society itself could be perfected. And that social perfection was, in fact, imperative as a way to usher in the one thousand years of peace that would preface Christ's final return to earth.

3. R. L. Numbers and R. C. Sawyer, "Medicine and Christianity in the Modern World," in *Health/Medicine and the Faith Traditions: An Enquiry into Religion and Medicine*, ed. Martin E. Marty and Kenneth L. Vaux (Philadelphia, 1982) 147.

4. For a comprehensive history of Catholic hospital care in the United States and its historical antecedents, see C. J. Kauffman, *Ministry and Meaning: A Religious History of Catholic Health Care in the United States* (New York, 1995).

5. The literature on Florence Nightingale is enormous. My sources for this and the following paragraphs are two standard biographies, Cecil Woodham-Smith's *Florence*

Nightingale (New York, 1951) and Mark Bostridge's *Florence Nightingale: The Woman and Her Legend* (New York, 2008).

6. See Mary Lindeman, *Medicine and Society in Early Modern Europe* (Cambridge, 2010) 188–92.

7. Information in this paragraph and the following paragraphs is from F. F. Cartwright, *A Social History of Medicine* (London, 1977) 151–54.

8. Against Foucault's views that definitions of madness were manufactured as an excuse for the confinement of society's deviants, see C. Jones and R. Porter, eds., *Reassessing Foucault: Power, Medicine, and the Body* (London, 1994).

9. For a short but comprehensive survey of Protestant medical missions in the nineteenth and twentieth centuries, see David Hardiman, introduction to *Healing Bodies, Saving Souls: Medical Missions in Asia and Africa*, ed. Hardiman (Amsterdam, 2006) 5–57. The volume contains several studies of Protestant missionary work during the past two centuries.

10. Numbers and Sawyer, "Medicine and Christianity" 149.

11. Ibid., 150.

12. Hardiman, introduction 15.

13. Numbers and Sawyer, "Medicine and Christianity" 151.

14. For a comprehensive history, see B. M. Wall, *Unlikely Entrepreneurs: Catholic Sisters and the Hospital Marketplace, 1865–1925* (Columbus, OH, 2005); and idem, *American Catholic Hospitals: A Century of Changing Markets and Missions* (Brunswick, NJ, 2011).

15. Kauffman, *Ministry and Meaning* 132.

16. M. R. O'Connell, "The Roman Catholic Tradition since 1545," in *Caring and Curing: Health and Medicine in the Western Religious Traditions*, ed. Ronald L. Numbers and Darrel W. Amundsen (1986; reprint, Baltimore, 1997) 136–37.

17. Numbers and Sawyer, "Medicine and Christianity" 139; D. W. Amundsen and G. B. Ferngren, "Epidemic Diseases," in *The History of Science and Religion in the Western Tradition: An Encyclopedia*, ed. G. B. Ferngren (New York, 2000) 491–94.

18. On the new emphasis on divine healing in North America in late nineteenth-century Protestantism, see H. D. Curtis, *Faith in the Great Physician: Suffering and Divine Healing in American Culture, 1860–1900* (Baltimore, 2007); and James Opp, *The Lord for the Body: Religion, Medicine, and Protestant Faith Healing in Canada, 1880–1930* (Montreal, 2005).

19. For a full description of the controversy and its religious and cultural background, see R. Ostrander, *The Life of Prayer in a World of Science: Protestants, Prayer, and American Culture, 1870–1930* (New York, 1999) 17–34; F. M. Turner, "Rainfall, Plagues, and the Prince of Wales," in *Contesting Cultural Authority: Essays in Victorian Intellectual Life* (Cambridge, 1993) 151–70; and R. B. Mullin, "Science, Miracles, and the Prayer-Gauge Debate," in *When Science and Christianity Meet*, ed. D. C. Lindberg and R. L. Numbers (Chicago, 2003) 203–24.

20. John Tyndall, "The 'Prayer for the Sick': Hints towards a Serious Attempt to Estimate Its Value," *Contemporary Review* 20 (1872), reprinted in *The Prayer-Gauge Debate* (Boston, 1876) 9–19.

21. Attempts scientifically to measure the efficacy of prayer in healing have continued

to the present. For a discussion of these attempts, see Claire Badaracco, *Prescribing Faith* (Waco, TX, 2007) 91–121.

22. On modernists' general rejection of petitionary prayer, for example, see Ostrander, *Life of Prayer*.

23. See P. Harrison, R. L. Numbers, and M. H. Shank, eds., *Wrestling with Nature: From Omens to Science* (Chicago, 2011).

24. See P. Starr, *The Social Transformation of American Medicine* (New York, 1982) 145–79.

25. Quoted in Numbers and Sawyer, "Medicine and Christianity" 137. See also C. E. Rosenberg and C. S. Rosenberg, "Pietism and the Origins of the American Public Health Movement: A Note on John H. Griscom and Robert M. Hartley," *Journal of the History of Medicine and Allied Sciences* 23 (1968): 16–35.

26. In referring to some Protestant American sects as "marginally Protestant," I mean to suggest that they are peripheral to a normative center in Protestantism. While their ecclesiology and outlook are Protestant, they owe their origins and distinctive doctrines to extrabiblical revelation by latter-day prophets that extend beyond conventional Protestant boundaries.

27. J. S. Haller Jr., *Sectarian Reformers in American Medicine, 1800–1910* (Brooklyn, NY, 2011) 56–57.

28. R. L. Numbers and D. R. Larson, "The Adventist Tradition," in Numbers and Amundsen, *Caring and Curing* 447–67.

29. W. H. Cumberland, "The Jehovah's Witness Tradition," in ibid., 468–85.

30. See R. L. Numbers and R. B. Schoepflin, "Ministries of Healing: Mary Baker Eddy, Ellen G. White, and the Religion of Health," in *Women and Health in America: A History*, ed. J. W. Leavitt (Madison, WI, 1984) 376–89.

31. R. B. Schoepflin, "The Christian Science Tradition," in Numbers and Amundsen, *Caring and Curing* 421–46. For a fuller treatment, see Schoepflin, *Christian Science on Trial: Religious Healing in America* (Baltimore, 2003).

32. See E. M. Umansky, *From Christian Science to Jewish Science: Spiritual Healing and American Jews* (New York, 2005).

33. L. E. Bush Jr., "The Mormon Tradition," in Numbers and Amundsen, *Caring and Curing* 400–405.

34. Ibid., 411, 414–15.

35. B. B. Warfield, *Counterfeit Miracles* (1918; reprint, London, 1972) 25–26.

36. On evolution in America, see R. L. Numbers, *Darwinism Comes to America* (Cambridge, MA, 1998). On biblical criticism, see Jerry Wayne Brown, *The Rise of Biblical Criticism in America, 1800–1870: The New England Scholars* (Middletown, CT, 1969); and Mark A. Noll, *Between Faith and Criticism: Evangelicals, Scholarship, and the Bible in America* (San Francisco, 1986). On secular influences, see Owen Chadwick, *The Secularism of the European Mind in the Nineteenth Century* (Cambridge, 1975).

37. See George M. Marsden, *Fundamentalism and American Culture: The Shaping of Twentieth Century Evangelicalism, 1870–1925* (New York, 1980). On the various meanings of fundamentalism in the 1920s, see Adam Laats, *Fundamentalism and Education in the Scopes Era: God, Darwin, and the Roots of America's Culture Wars* (Basingstoke, UK, 2010).

38. Pamela Klassen describes the attraction that alternative healing methods had for

Canadian theological liberals in the United and Anglican Churches, who, in rejecting orthodox Christianity, sought modes of religious healing that reflected the modern age, many of them not rational. P. E. Klassen, *Spirits of Protestantism: Medicine, Healing, and Liberal Christianity* (Berkeley and Los Angeles, 2011).

39. On the history of the eugenics movement in the South, see E. J. Larson, *Sex, Race, and Science: Eugenics in the Deep South* (Baltimore, 1995). On its decline in the South, see ibid., 149–64 and 168. Some American eugenicists praised the Nazi program (see ibid., 147).

40. For the most recent treatment of the origins of Pentecostalism, see R. J. Stephens, *The Fire Spreads: The Origins of Holiness and Pentecostalism in the American South* (Cambridge, MA, 2008).

41. See E. L. Blumhofer, *Aimee Semple McPherson: Everybody's Sister* (Grand Rapids, MI, 1993).

42. See David Harrel, *Oral Roberts: An American Life* (Bloomington, IN, 1985).

43. A movement that encouraged sacramental healing arose among Anglo-Catholics in Britain in the 1920s. Services of healing are often held today in Anglican and Episcopal churches.

44. On "Lourdes water" and American replicas of the grotto at Lourdes, see C. McDannell, "Lourdes Water and American Catholicism," in *Material Christianity: Religion and Popular Culture in America* (New Haven, CT, 1995) 132–62. On Lourdes, see Ruth Harris's sympathetic portrayal, with a personal statement in her preface (xiii–xviii), *Lourdes: Body and Spirit in the Secular Age* (New York, 1999).

45. See Sergio Luzzatto, *Padre Pio* (Turin, Italy, 2007). For a detailed study of canonization, see J. Duffin, *Medical Miracles: Doctors, Saints, and Healing in the Modern World* (Oxford, 2009). Duffin offers a revealing personal statement of how a modern critical historian approaches religious miracles of healing (183–90).

46. See Robert A. Orsi, "'Mildred, Is It Fun to Be a Cripple?': The Culture of Suffering in Mid-Twentieth Century American Catholicism," *South Atlantic Quarterly* 93 (1994): 547–90.

47. Eliot N. Dorff, "The Jewish Tradition," in Numbers and Amundsen, *Caring and Curing* 7.

48. Ibid., 7–8; N. J. Zohar, "The Discourses of Jewish Medical Ethics," in *The Cambridge World History of Medical Ethics*, ed. Robert B. Baker and Laurence B. McCullough (New York, 2009) 267–68. On how Halakhic support is applied to such modern issues as artificial insemination by a donor and to euthanasia, see N. Solomon, "From Folk Medicine to Bioethics in Judaism," in *Religion, Health and Suffering*, ed. John R. Hinnels and Roy Porter (London, 1999) 176–81.

49. See Immanuel Jakobovits, *Jewish Medical Ethics: A Comparative and Historical Study of the Jewish Religious Attitude to Medicine and Its Practice* (New York, 1975), esp. 251–94.

50. See Cathy Siebold, *The Hospice Movement: Easing Death's Pains* (New York, 1992), esp. 1–27, for a brief historical background. The term *palliative care* was first popularized in 1975. The story of Hospice is told in Shirley du Boulay, *Cicely Saunders: The Founder of the Modern Hospice Movement* (London, 1984); see esp. 85–102.

51. See W. Cadge, *Paging God: Religion in the Halls of Medicine* (Chicago, 2012), for a comprehensive history of hospital chaplaincy.

52. A. M. van Loon, "Faith Community (Parish) Nursing," in *Oxford Textbook of Spirituality in Healthcare*, ed. M. Cobb, C. M. Puchalski, and B. Rumbold (Oxford, 2012) 219–26.

53. See O'Connell, "The Roman Catholic Tradition since 1545" 140.

54. See T. L. Beauchamp and J. F. Childress, *Principles of Bioethics* (New York, 2001), for discussions of these and other issues in bioethics from a Catholic perspective.

55. On the history of Catholic views of contraception, see J. T. Noonan Jr., *Contraception: A History of Its Treatment by the Catholic Theologians and Canonists* (Cambridge, MA, 1986).

56. Paul VI requested that the commission address whether the newly developed anovular pill was licit. For the pre-conciliar trajectory that culminated in *Humanae vitae*, see Leslie Tentler, *Catholics and Contraception: An American History* (Ithaca, NY, 2004).

57. O'Connell, "Roman Catholic Tradition Since 1545" 141; Bernard Häring, "The Encyclical Crisis," *Commonweal* 88 (1968): 588, quoted in D. W. Amundsen, "The Discourses of Roman Catholic Medical Ethics," in Baker and McCullough, *Cambridge World History of Medical Ethics* 236.

58. Amundsen, "Discourses of Roman Catholic Medical Ethics" 235–37.

59. A. Verhey and S. E. Lammers, eds., *Theological Voices in Medical Ethics* (Grand Rapids, MI, 1993) 7–29.

60. Ibid., 106–26; William F. May, *The Physician's Covenant: Images of the Healer in Medical Ethics* (Philadelphia, 1983).

61. See Verhey and Lammers, *Theological Voices* 600–611. Biblical passages often cited include, for example, Jer. 1:5, Ps. 139:15–16, and Lk 1:41 on abortion.

62. G. Ferngren, "The Imago Dei and the Sanctity of Life: The Origins of an Idea," in *Euthanasia and the Newborn: Conflicts Regarding Saving Lives*, ed. R. C. McMillan, H. Tristram Engelhardt Jr., and S. F. Spicker (Dordrecht, 1987) 23–45.

63. G. Ferngren, "The Evangelical-Fundamentalist Tradition," in Numbers and Amundsen, *Caring and Curing* 504–5.

64. See E. J. Larson and D. W. Amundsen, *A Different Death: Euthanasia and the Christian Tradition* (Downers Grove, IL, 1998).

65. Ferngren, "Evangelical-Fundamentalist Tradition" 505–7.

66. S. E. Lammers and A. Verhey, eds., *On Moral Medicine: Theological Perspectives in Medical Ethics* (Grand Rapids, MI, 1998) 655–62, 671–78.

67. C. S. Campbell, "Religious Views on Biotechnology, Protestant," in *Encyclopedia of Ethical, Legal, and Policy Issues in Biotechnology*, ed. Thomas J. Murray and Maxwell J. Mehlmen (New York, 2000) 938–47.

68. J. M. Gustafson, *Protestant and Roman Catholic Ethics: Prospects for Rapprochement* (Chicago, 1978) 126–37.

69. Keith Thomas, *Man and the Natural World: Changing Attitudes in England, 1500–1800* (London, 1983) 173–91. Thomas terms the animal-rights tradition "latent in the Judaeo-Christian tradition" (181).

70. On the secularization of medical ethics, see John Evans, *Playing God* (Chicago, 2002).

71. S. J. Sutcliffe, *Children of the New Age: A History of Spiritual Practices* (London, 2003) 174–94.

72. The term *holism* was coined by the South African statesman and philosopher Jan Smuts (1870–1950) in his *Holism and Evolution* (London, 1926). Vitalism is the view that the body is animated by a life force.

73. See E. Baruman, A. I. Brint, L. Piper, and P. A. Wright, eds., *The Holistic Health Handbook: A Tool for Attaining Wholeness of Body, Mind, and Spirit* (Berkeley, 1981).

74. For the relationship between traditional and alternative medicines, see B. Inglis, *Natural Medicine* (Glasgow, 1979).

75. Tracy Fessenden's argument that secularization in the United States is in fact the successful dissemination of a pan-Protestant ethos is widely accepted as an authoritative reading of American "secularization." See Fessenden, *Culture and Redemption: Religion, the Secular, and American Literature* (Princeton, NJ, 2007). See also Ronald Numbers, who argues that supernatural religion has "not only persisted but flourished" in modern Western societies in spite of the cultural dominance of science, but that religious views have been pushed out of the public sphere and into the private, where they continue to enjoy a healthy existence even among a minority of practicing scientists, who are no less religious than were many scientists a century ago. Numbers, "Science, Secularization, and Privatization," in *Science and Christianity in Pulpit and Pew* (New York, 2007) 29–136, quotation from 129.

EPILOGUE

1. See Noel Annan, "Historismus and History," in *Our Age: English Intellectuals between the World Wars—A Group Portrait* (New York, 1990) 263–79.

2. Cf. Helen King, "Medicine," in *A Companion to Ancient History*, ed. Andrew Erskine (Chichester, UK, 2009) 403.

3. The phrase, better known in its modified Latin translation, is found in the Hippocratic treatise *Epidemics*, bk. 1, sec. 11.

4. Strictly speaking, theodicy attempts to account for suffering in a religion characterized by belief in a deity that is both good and all-powerful. On the place of suffering in diverse medical and faith traditions, see John R. Hinnels and Roy Porter, eds., *Religion, Health and Suffering* (London, 1999).

5. O. Zöcker, quoted in F. Scott Spencer, "2 Chronicles 28:5–15 and the Parable of the Good Samaritan," *Westminster Theological Journal* 46 (1984): 319.

6. From a Latin antiphon attributed to Notker, "The Stammerer," a monk of St. Gall, in 911. It has been incorporated into the service at the grave in The Order for the Burial of the Dead in the Book of Common Prayer (1928 American revision).

7. For a poignant account of a family whose refusal to administer insulin for their son's diabetes on religious grounds led to his death, see Larry Parker, *We Let Our Son Die: A Parent's Search for Truth* (Eugene, OR, 1980).

8. Albert Camus, *The Plague*, trans. Stuart Gilbert (New York, 1948), originally published as *La Peste* in 1947.

9. Ibid., 89.

10. I owe my comparison of Father Paneloux's two sermons to Bernard Ramm, *The Devil, Seven Wormwoods, and God* (Waco, TX, 1977) 101–3.

11. Laurie Zoloth, "The Duty of Repair in a Broken World: Ethical Issues in Medical Research" (paper, First Conference on Medicine and Religion, Chicago, May 2012) 3. The paper draws on the ideas of the Lithuanian French philosopher of Judaism, Emmanel Levinas.

Index